All About Osteoarthritis

All About Osteoarthritis

The Definitive Resource
for Arthritis Patients and Their Families

NANCY E. LANE AND DANIEL J. WALLACE

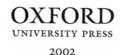

OXFORD
UNIVERSITY PRESS
2002

OXFORD
UNIVERSITY PRESS

Oxford New York
Auckland Bangkok
Buenos Aires Cape Town Chennai Dar es Salaam Delhi
Hong Kong Istanbul Karachi Kolkata
Kuala Lumpur Madrid Melbourne
Mexico City Mumbai Nairobi São Paulo Shanghai
Singapore Taipei Tokyo Toronto

and associated companies in Berlin

Published by Oxford University Press, Inc.
198 Madison Avenue, New York, New York 10016

Oxford is a registered trademark of Oxford University Press

Library of Congress Cataloging-in-Publication Data
Lane, Nancy E.
All about osteoarthritis / Nancy E. Lane and Daniel J. Wallace.
p.   cm.
Includes bibliographical references and index.
ISBN 0-19-513873-2
1. Osteoarthritis—Popular works.
I. Wallace, Daniel J. (Daniel Jeffrey), 1949–
II. Title.

RC931 .O67 L36 2001
616.7'223—dc21   2001036143

Illustrations by Teri A. Hoffman

1 3 5 7 9 8 6 4 2

Printed in the United States of America
on acid-free paper

Contents

Contents

Preface

All About Osteoarthritis represents the sixth in a successful series of books covering rheumatic disease related topics including lupus, fibromyalgia, scleroderma, osteoporosis, and Sjogren's syndrome. In 1995, Oxford University Press pioneered the concept of reviewing important medical topics for lay people, allied health professionals, and physicians. Prior to that time, there existed a gap between literature disseminated by disease-oriented foundations and medical textbooks where one could not obtain a detailed, readable, concise, and medically accurate review of rheumatic disease topics. We are encouraged to have the support of the National Osteoporosis Foundation, Arthritis Foundation, Lupus Foundation of America, Scleroderma Foundation, and Sjorgren's Syndrome Foundation. Osteoarthritis is an extremely common, poorly understood, under-researched disorder. It has been an exciting challenge attempting to distill voluminous facts and information into this text. The reader will judge how successful our efforts were. The authors are grateful to the assistance provided by UCLA medical artist Terri Hoffman, Cedars-Sinai radiologist Douglas Brown, M.D., Oxford editors Joan Bossert, Janice Wallace, Fred M. Tileston and all other family members (Trevor Tileston, Reid Tileston).

Nancy E. Lane and Daniel J. Wallace
San Francisco and Los Angeles, 2001

All About Osteoarthritis

Part 1

INTRODUCTION
AND DEFINITIONS

Arthritis is a general pain of all the joints; that of the feet we call Podagara; that of the hip joint, Schiatica; that of the hand, Chiagra . . . Arthritis fixes itself . . . sometimes in the hip-joints; and for the most part in these cases, the patient remains lame on it.

—Arataeus the Cappadocian (81–138 A.D.)
On Arthritis and Schiatica

Patients come to us all the time and implore, "Doc, can't you do something about my arthritis?" All too often, arthritis is viewed as a single disorder. In fact, arthritis represents over 150 separate conditions divided into at least 7 different broad categories, or "families." This section will explore what arthritis is and how concepts of it evolved historically. We will begin to focus on osteoarthritis specifically, define terms, and start to explore who develops the disorder.

Introduction

Why Write a Book about Osteoarthritis?

Few things are so apt to cause a drowsy despair at a medical meeting as the prospect of an academic discussion on . . . osteoarthritis. The field is so barren, the harvest is small . . .
—John Kent Spender (1829–1916),
in the *British Medical Journal*, 1888

In medical school many years ago, the professor who introduced the musculoskeletal system to one of us referred to osteoarthritis as a disorder where "patients never died and never got better." This flippant remark belied the enormity of a problem which threatens to overwhelm organized medicine's ability to marshall resources to deal with osteoarthritis in the twenty-first century.

Among the 150 rheumatic disorders classified and characterized by the Arthritis Foundation, osteoarthritis is the most common. It accounts for 60 percent of the patients and visits to physicians with musculoskeletal complaints. Forty-three million Americans have symptomatic and clinically relevant arthritis, and 6 million of those afflicted have never seen a physician. According to the American Medical Association, every day 23% of the United States population complain of joint pain, 22% suffer from backache, 21% have sore feet, 20% experience muscle pain, and 18% have arthritis discomfort.

The consequences of society's benign neglect of osteoarthritis is staggering:

3

1. The management of 23 million Americans with osteoarthritis and related disorders costs 149 billion dollars a year in indirect and direct costs and constitutes 2.5% of our gross national product.
2. Patients with osteoarthritis record 315 million doctor visits per year.
3. Osteoarthritis is responsible in some way for 744,000 hospitalizations a year, representing 4 million days of in-patient care, and is listed as an associated diagnosis for another 8 million hospital admissions.
4. Though two-thirds of people older than 65 years of age have osteoarthritis, 44% with the disease are under 65, and it affects 12.1% of the United States population over the age of 25.
5. Osteoarthritis is responsible for 68 million days of missed work every year, and results in losses of 95 billion dollars in lost wages and medical costs and another 1.5 billion from restricted work activities.
6. Osteoarthritis is the second most common cause of disability (and most common after the age of 65) in the United States. About 5% of the work force retires due to osteoarthritis each year.
7. Although 300,000 hip and knee surgeries are performed each year in the United States, 100,000 Americans cannot walk independently from their bed to their bathroom due to hip or knee osteoarthritis.
8. By the year 2020, 60 million Americans will have arthritis (half, or 30 million, of whom will have osteoarthritis). This represents an aging population which will increase disability costs by 25%.

What are the possible results of this public health nightmare? First, the average osteoarthritis patient spends $2,650 a year on his/her care, and knows little about his/her disorder. According to a study at Stanford University, a self-help educational course on managing arthritis can decrease physician visits by half and pain perception by 20%. Over 60% of osteoarthritis patients use unproven, over-the-counter remedies for arthritis on a regular basis. Desperate conditions lead to desperate measures, most of which is the fault of suboptimal organized rheumatic disease advocacy. Osteoarthritis impairs work, leisure activities, shopping, household chores, marriage, family enjoyment, sexuality, and ultimately one's ability to be independent. Though more common than stroke or circulatory disorders, osteoarthritis benefits from much less research focus or attention.

How can this book make a difference? Although Amazon.com lists 73 books under the keyword "osteoarthritis," fewer than 5 were written by rheumatologists for osteoarthritis patients. To our knowledge, ours is the only one currently in print written by active investigators in the field for patients, primary care physicians, and allied health professionals. With this book the patient will learn what osteoarthritis is, how to help themselves, and how to find the best resources to manage the disorder. We will also outline recent advances in the field, and discuss where these breakthroughs will lead us.

1

What Is Osteoarthritis?

A definition is the enclosing a wilderness of idea within a wall of words.

—Samuel Butler (d. 1902),
"Higgeldy-Piggeldy," *Note Books* (1912)

The word "arthritis," meaning "inflammation of a joint," is a misnomer. Many rheumatic conditions do not inflame joints, and some do not even involve the joints at all. Our body has 640 muscles, 212 bones, and 100 joints. Just about anything can go wrong with any of them.

THE FAMILIES OF ARTHRITIS

The family of osteoarthritis is the subject of this book. Table 1 lists the 7 families, which include 90% of the 150 rheumatic disorders recognized by the American College of Rheumatology. Some of the other types of arthritis (which we prefer to call rheumatic diseases) are categorized as follows: *crystal arthritis* (mostly due to gout—a uric acid crystal or pseudogout, which is a calcium pyrophosphate crystal): *septic arthritis* (due to an infection in a joint such as staphlococcus, or a musculoskeletal reaction to an infection as in rheumatic fever or Lyme disease); *autoimmune disorders* (including lupus or rheumatoid arthritis); *soft tissue conditions* which spare the joints (such as fibromyalgia or bursitis); *disorders of bone modeling* (too much calcium in bone causes osteopetrosis,

Table 1: The spectrum of arthritis—7 groups and their prevalence in the United States

---

- Osteoarthritis (23 million)
- Crystal induced arthritis (3 million)
- Rheumatoid variant/reactive arthritis (1 million)
- Metabolic bone disease (20 million)
- Autoimmune rheumatic disease/ rheumatoid arthritis (3 million)
- Septic arthritis (less than 1 million)
- Soft tissue rheumatism (includes everybody at some time)

while too little results in osteoporosis); and *rheumatoid variants* (the arthritis of inflammatory bowel disease, ankylosing spondylitis, and reactive arthritis). Osteoarthritis can coexist with these conditions as well.

COMING TO TERMS: HOW DO WE DEFINE OSTEOARTHRITIS?

Osteoarthritis, also referred to as degenerative joint disease, is a form of arthritis that results from degeneration of the articular cartilage in the joint. As we will discuss in chapter 5, articular cartilage is like a sponge that covers the ends of bones when they meet the joint—for example, where the femur (thigh bone) and the tibia (shin bone) meet at the knee. The main function of articular cartilage is to be a shock absorber or cushion in the joint. It is also a slippery material that allows the joints to slide back and forth with very little friction. Osteoarthritis or joint degeneration occurs when the articular cartilage wears out, or is worn down so that it works much less efficiently. When the cartilage wears out, it decreases in size or volume. Without cartilage or with less cartilage, bones lose their shock-absorbing buffers and begin to rub against each other. For example, with osteoarthritis of the knee, joint pain develops when you walk because the cartilage is not able to provide shock absorption. As the disease progresses, changes also occur in the muscles and bones around the joints with osteoarthritis. However, the primary problem in osteoarthritis is degeneration of the articular cartilage, and over time people develop pain in their joints when they use them, as well as joint stiffness and joint swelling. The most common joints to develop osteoarthritis are the hips, knees, back, neck, and hands, but the process can occur in almost any joint.

Since osteoarthritis results from the loss of articular cartilage, it is often referred to as a "wear and tear" disease. This is not exactly true since one does not always have to injure a joint to develop osteoarthritis. However, osteoarthritis does develop at a more rapid rate in individuals who have injured cartilage in the knee. While the mechanical basis of the disease is the major abnormality, there is also a biochemical element. We will discuss this in chapters 5 and 6. Also, some osteoarthritis may have hereditary basis.

SUMMARY

Osteoarthritis results from degeneration or "wearing out" of the articular cartilage in joints. It commonly causes pain when the joint is used. There are many reasons for cartilage to degenerate, and both mechanical and biochemical factors cause osteoarthritis.

2

The History of Osteoarthritis

It is not disgraceful that a person should, by reason of that extraordinary thing arthritis, be unable to use his hands and should need somebody to bring food to his mouth for him . . . One cannot overlook the pain these people suffer, night and day, as though their maladies were torturers twisting them on the rack . . .

—Galen (128–200 A.D.)

Although arthritis was mentioned by scholars in ancient Greece and Rome, such as Hippocrates and Galen, its differentiation into distinct disorders did not take place until the nineteenth century. By the late 1800s, "chronic arthritis" was divided into "atrophic" and "hypertrophic" components. Atrophic disease included several conditions now associated with inflammation of the synovium, and erosion or atrophy of cartilage and bone. This category consisted of rheumatoid arthritis, ankylosing spondylitis, and gout. Hypertrophic disease was coined due to its "excess growth," or hypertrophy of adjacent bone and soft tissues. John Kent Spender of Bath, England, was the first to use the term "osteoarthritis" to denote hypertrophic arthritis in 1886. Clinical evaluation methods which could distinguish it from rheumatoid-like arthritis were widely accepted by the first decade of the twentieth century largely due to efforts by Archibald E. Garrod of London.

The hallmark nodules found in the hands of osteoarthritis patients are named after William Hebreden (who described those found in the

9

distal knuckles in 1802) and Charles Bouchard who described involvement of the middle knuckles in 1884). The formation of the International League Against Rheumatism and the evolution of the forerunners of the Arthritis Foundation and the American College of Rheumatology in the late 1920s and 1930s, along with efforts by the Royal Society of Medicine in England, led to several nomenclature classifications of arthritis which accurately defined and classified osteoarthritis. In the late 1940s and early 1950s, Jonas Kellgren was the first to detail X-ray abnormalities associated with osteoarthritis, as well as delineating some of its subsets (erosive, inflammatory, and generalized).

People have attempted to alleviate arthritis suffering with mixed success for thousands of years. Stone tablets from the Sumerian period confirmed that the Assyrians used the extract of willow leaves to treat arthritis, as did the ancient Egyptians and Greeks. The first scientific exploration of willow bark extract therapy for musculoskeletal pain was published by Reverend Edmund Stone from Chipping Norton, Oxfordshire in 1763. Various iterations of European willow bark evolved into what we know now as aspirin, primarily due to efforts by Bayer and Company in Germany between 1874 and 1899. Derivatives of acetaminophen, another agent which had analgesic properties, ultimately led to the introduction of what we know now popularly as Tylenol in 1948. Modifications of aspirin led to the introduction of the first nonsteroidal anti-inflammatory drug (NSAID), phenylbutazone, in the early 1950s. Ibuprofen, naproxen, and others soon became widely available. Side effects, which were primarily gastrointestinal, precluded the American College of Rheumatology from recommending them for osteoarthritis until 2000, when selective "cox-2" inhibitors (e.g., rofecoxib, known by the brand name Vioxx, and the celecoxib in Celebrex) received not only FDA approval for osteoarthritis but the college's endorsement.

The formation of the American Academy of Orthopedic Surgeons in 1933 sowed the seeds of intellectual curiousity which led to dramatic advances in joint replacement surgery. The introduction of anesthesia (1846), aseptic surgery (1865), X-rays (1895), and antibiotics (1939) provided the foundation for successful orthopedic procedures. The first use of biocompatible materials by Charles Venable and Walter Stuck in 1938 allowed for the first modern successful hip replacement in 1939. We have clearly come a long way, but our management of osteoarthritis is still in its infancy and in need of new creative strategies, ingenuity, and wisdom.

3

Who Gets Osteoarthritis?

Diseases may . . . color moods of civilizations.
—René Dubos (1901–1982)
Man, Medicine & Environment (1968)

Osteoarthritis, has existed as far back as the prehistoric eras—it has been found in dinosaur skeletons, and affects all mammals. Studies of skeleton X-rays from all ages show that if one lives long enough, osteoarthritis will develop in some joints. However, even though more than 80% of X-rays in people older than 75 years have osteoarthritis of the knee, less than 30% of people will ever develop knee pain from their osteoarthritis. Other estimates are that 10–15% of all Americans suffer from osteoarthritis knee pain. Clearly there is a large discrepancy between those that have X-ray evidence of osteoarthritis and those who eventually develop joint pain; however, the reasons for this are not yet clear.

The older we get, the higher the chance of getting osteoarthritis, with a nearly 90% chance of X-ray findings in some joint by age 75. However, after the seventh decade the incidence appears to plateau, and this may mean that those who reach this age without symptoms are not likely to get them or that it has not yet been carefully studied in older individuals. While osteoarthritis appears to be an inescapable cause of aging, there is still no clear link between the normal aging process and the articular cartilage loss seen with osteoarthritis. Here we will review the risk factors for developing osteoarthritis (summarized in Table 3, at the end of the section).

PEOPLE WHO ARE ABOVE WEIGHT
DEVELOP OSTEOARTHRITIS

Overweight women are about nine times more likely to develop osteoarthritis than women of normal weight, and overweight men are four times more likely than normal weight men. In general, more weight increases loading on the joints, such as the hips and knees, and may accelerate joint degeneration. When the Center for Disease Control (CDC) surveyed 25,000 Americans over the age of 25, they discovered that the association between body weight and osteoarthritis becomes stronger when people become heavier. As shown in Table 2, researchers divided weights into six categories: underweight, normal weight, above weight, and 3 increasing levels of weight. In addition, Body Mass Index (BMI = height in meters divided by weight in kilograms) was used to determine the different levels. For example, men five feet ten inches tall and of normal weight (129–173 pounds) have about a 3% risk for osteoarthritis; above that weight (174–208) men ran a 4% risk; as the obesity level increased, the percentages jumped to about 5%, and 6%, and at the highest level of weight (277 pounds) to 10%. Women five feet five inches and at normal weight (111–149 pounds) had a 5% osteoarthritis risk; overweight or mild obesity (150–179 pounds) were at 9%; and the heaviest level (more than 270 pounds) was at 17%. This large population-based study is one of many showing that in both women and men, increased weight is associated with a greater risk for developing osteoarthritis.

Table 2: Prevalence of osteoarthritis by body mass index (kg/m²) — a survey of 17,000 Americans >25 years of age

Category	Men (%)	Women (%)
Underweight	0.4	0.8
Normal weight	2.6	5.2
Above weight	4.4	8.5
Mild obesity	4.7	9.4
Moderate obesity	5.5	10.4
Severe obesity	10.6	17.2

*   Men = 67", 129–173 lbs; women, 65", 111–149 lbs.

WOMEN ARE MORE SUSCEPTIBLE TO OSTEOARTHRITIS

Women develop osteoarthritis about twice as often as men. Age is a factor—men under 45 years have more symptoms than women, and it is about the same for men and women between 45–55 years. After the age of 55, women appear more likely to develop the disease. There are some areas of the body that differ in frequencies between the genders. Women are much more likely to develop osteoarthritis of the fingers and hand than men, and men develop hip osteoarthritis at a younger age than women.

Since osteoarthritis of the hands and knees is very common in women and osteoarthritis of the hand usually appears just after menopause in women, researchers have focused their attention on estrogen and its relationship to osteoarthritis in women. In laboratory studies estrogen has had some positive effects on cartilage, but studies in animal models of osteorthritis have not found estrogen to be protective of cartilage. Also, clinical studies that have examined associations of estrogen and osteoarthritis have found only that having children provides a small protective effect, and no effect was found for estrogen levels at menopause or age of menopause. Estrogen use may prevent the development of osteoarthritis, but there is no evidence that it slows the progression of the disease. The role of estrogen in the management of osteoarthritis is reviewed in chapter 18.

IS OSTEOARTHRITIS MORE PREVALENT IN RACIAL OR ETHNIC GROUPINGS?

In almost all races and ethnic groups, osteoarthritis develops and has a high prevalence in the elderly. However, there is some evidence that Asians, especially Chinese, have lower rates of hip but higher rates of knee osteoarthritis. African-American men and women tend to have higher rates of osteoarthritis than other races. These different rates for developing osteoarthritis may reflect genetic, socioeconomic, and lifestyle factors. Much more research is needed in this area.

IS THERE A ROLE FOR GENES AND HEREDITY?

There are a number of studies performed in identical twins and nonidentical or fraternal twins demonstrating that osteoarthritis—

especially of the hand, hip, and knee—has a high heritable component, ranging from 40–65%. In addition to inheriting genes that generate incorrectly working proteins, which cause cartilage to wear out, we inherit other parts of the musculoskeletal system that increase our risk of developing osteoarthritis. Collagen, a protein that makes up most of the ligaments can be weak from inheriting an abnormal collagen gene: weak ligaments increase stress on the joints.

An example of weak collagen in the ligaments is referred to as an "Ehler-Danlos" variant, or double-jointedness. People who are double-jointed can stretch their elbows out more than 180 degrees, and pop their thumbs out of their joints. Sometimes they dislocate their kneecap or patella, because the ligaments are too weak to hold it in place. Individuals with weak collagen can sometimes even stretch their knees back so that the calf muscle sits behind the knee. We inherit a copy of a gene from each parent, and most people with evidence of Ehler-Danlos syndrome are "heterozygotes"—instead of receiving two good genes they have one good gene and one abnormal copy (or allele), with the result that their collagen is about 50% weaker than that of a normal person. When someone inherits two copies of abnormal collagen genes, they have even more problems with their joints and their ligaments may be too weak to support the body while walking. These people are very disabled.

Another type of osteoarthritis with a high inheritable potential is in the hand—where one can develop "knobby knuckles," or Heberden's and Bouchard's nodes. This type of osteoarthritis is found in families, and women are more affected than men. One study found that about 50% of children inherited Heberden's nodes from their parents and there was a suggestion that the disease was more severe when developed at an earlier age.

In all likelihood, there are a large number of genes that contribute to the development of osteoarthritis. Defects in the genes that cause the disease may be in the components that make up the articular cartilage—proteoglycans, collagen type II, other proteins and sugars, or components of bone near the joints. A few years ago, a research group in Ohio described a family that developed osteoarthritis of the hips, knees, and ankles in early adulthood. Isolation of the gene for collagen type II in the affected family members revealed that the genes for this protein had an abnormal allele coding for an animo acid. When this incorrect amino acid was put into the collagen, the collagen was weak and led to osteoarthritis at a very early age. The identification of this abnormal gene product in the collagen type II was a major breakthrough. It was recognized in this family because osteoarthritis tended to develop in weight-bearing joints about 30 years before expected. Premature development of the disease led physicians to consider a genetic defect or inherited genetic trait that predisposed the patients to this disease so early.

Researchers have also reported a genetic association between radiographic osteoarthritis and the insulin growth factor—(IGF-1) gene. The IGF-1 protein stimulates cells in the cartilage to make more cartilage. If someone makes too little IGF-1, they may not replace cartilage, and thus over time develop osteoarthritis. It is also possible to make too much IGF-1 (or have an abnormal IGF-1 protein), and in this case, cartilage may be replaced too often, rendering it weak.

This discussion is meant to raise awareness that common diseases such as osteoarthritis can have a strong genetic component. Already researchers have identified a predisposition to osteoarthritis as a result of abnormally functioning proteins, and in the next few years there will most likely be hundreds of new genetic associations with osteoarthritis. We will find a number of genes that code for abnormal proteins in individuals who develop osteoarthritis at an early age or have a rapid progression of their disease. Some of the genes associated with osteoarthritis will have large effects (such as the defective protein produced in collagen type II) or minor effects, such as the abnormal collagen produced in someone who is double-jointed, or has "ligamentous laxity." Piecing this puzzle together will answer thousands of questions about this very common disease.

JOINT "WEAR AND TEAR" CAUSES OSTEOARTHRITIS: TRUTH OR MYTH?

For many years it was commonly believed that if you used your joints a lot, they would "wear out" sooner than if you did not use them. Since osteoarthritis was referred to as a disease of "wear and tear," this seemed logical.

To determine if joints wore out and developed osteoarthritis sooner with high use, we devised a study comparing middle-aged runners with a mean age of 55, who were running about 30 miles a week for over 9 years, to a community control group of men who were generally not runners. We performed physical examinations, obtained X-rays of knees, spines, and hands, and bone density measurements of the spine on all of the study subjects. The runners had no evidence of increased radiographic and clinical osteoarthritis compared to the control group. However, we did find that the runners appeared to have a better overall health status and higher bone mass in the spine. We continued to follow the groups for over 10 years, and during that time, knee osteoarthritis developed in a few runners and a few controls—but even after 10 more years of running or jogging, there was no increased incidence of knee osteoarthritis. We concluded from this study that while not everyone who is middle-aged can run or jog (and individuals that have osteoarthritis already—or painful joints—would not have been in the running group), individuals with normal knee joints can probably run forever without increasing their risk of developing knee osteoarthritis. As individuals age, however, running and jogging does not always "feel good" and many runners and joggers become brisk walkers or turn to other types of exercise. After 10 years, even if some of the runners were no longer running, they still were in better health, overall, than those in the nonrunning control group. In summary, then, heavy joint use of normal joints does not accelerate the development of osteoarthritis even in middle aged and elderly runners—unless there is previous joint injury.

WHAT ABOUT A HISTORY OF JOINT INJURY?

Unfortunately, individuals who injure a joint, especially a weight-bearing knee joint, are at increased risk for developing osteoarthritis in that affected joint. The types of injuries to the internal structures in the knee includes the cartilage (the menisci), the ligaments within the knee (anterior cruciate ligament), or around the knee (medial and lateral collateral ligaments). In a study of ex-elite runners in Finland, the risk of knee osteoarthritis was increased several fold for those runners who had a history of knee injury compared to other athletes who did not run. In a study in Sweden of middle-aged adult soccer players, a previous knee injury increased the risk of developing knee osteoarthritis several fold compared to soccer players who had not injured their knees. Another study in England found that a history of surgery for a meniscal repair or its partial removal increased the risk of knee osteoarthritis in athletes. The disease developed in less than 9 years in athletes who sustained the injury and had surgical removal of the torn meniscus after the age of 20 and took 20 years to develop if the injury was sustained before age 20. In a study of middle-aged runners and community controls that we performed at Stanford beginning in 1984, a history of knee injury also increased the risk of knee osteoarthritis several fold compared to the community controls.

It is clear that sports injuries increase the risk for the development of osteoarthritis in the affected joint. Studies also find that the older one is when the joint is injured, the faster osteoarthritis develops. The risk of developing osteoarthritis in the affected joint increases even if surgery is performed to repair the torn cartilage or torn ligament. This is the result of abnormal biomechanics that occur despite repair of the injuries.

Arthritis resulting from joint injury is referred to as *secondary* osteoarthritis, as the joint injury provides a cause for joint degeneration. When osteoarthritis develops without an underlying cause, it is referred to as *primary* or *idiopathic* osteoarthritis.

Osteoarthritis resulting from sporting injuries is on the rise, as more people are exercising and playing sports in their leisure time. Individuals tend to start exercise or recreational activity in young adulthood, and these activities might continue for over 30 years. The long-term impact upon the risk of developing osteoarthritis is just now beginning to be studied. For example, Caucasian women were asked about their recreational activities from their teenage years through age 50; those who exercised regularly as a teenager were about twice as likely to develop hip osteoarthritis compared to similar control groups that did not exercise. Therefore, while these studies must be interpreted with caution, we know that physical activities in middle age do not accelerate the development of osteoarthritis, while sports that begin in the teenage years and are continued may over a long period of time have a detrimental effect on the joints. More studies will need to be done to determine if longer-term physical activity predisposes us to joint degeneration.

WHAT WORK ACTIVITIES OR OCCUPATIONS INCREASE OSTEOARTHRITIS RISKS?

Certain types of occupations that put high stress on different parts of the skeleton can increase the risk for developing osteoarthritis in the hip and knee. Although not much research has been done, one study showed that occupations involving repeated kneeling, squatting, heavy lifting, or stair-climbing were associated with an increased risk of knee osteoarthritis. In England, a study found that farmers run a higher risk of developing hip osteoarthritis than individuals that do not farm. Jack-hammer drivers, cotton pickers, and bus drivers have also been found to have more hand osteoarthritis than other professions. These studies suggest that some activities, when done repeatedly for a number of years, accelerate joint degeneration. Again, abnormal loads to normal joints over time probably increases the risk of developing osteoarthritis in that joint. Most likely, working in some occupations—together with other risk factors for osteoarthritis, such as age or being overweight— also play a major role in the development of osteoarthritis and the pain and disability that is associated with it.

CAN VITAMIN DEFICIENCY CAUSE OSTEOARTHRITIS?

Over the last few years, we have come to understand that cartilage is con-tinually renewed, and its breakdown and replacement can be influenced by a number of vitamins and minerals. Some population-based studies have reported that low blood levels of vitamin D increase the risk for de-velopment of hip osteoarthritis, and the progression of knee osteoarthri-tis is about twofold compared to individuals with normal serum levels of this vitamin. Since vitamin D is known to prevent enzymes from being activated that break down cartilage, it may be that individuals with low vi-tamin D levels increase their enzyme levels and break down cartilage more quickly. Others studies have found that the fat soluble vitamins A and E, and water soluble vitamin C, may also slow the breakdown of carti-lage because they have anti-oxidative properties that may protect cartilage against breakdown. Despite this new evidence that low levels of vitamins in the bloodstream may accelerate cartilage breakdown, the current rec-ommendation for normal daily adult doses of these vitamins has not changed. There have been no clinical studies that have found that high dose replacement of these vitamins alters the course of osteoarthritis.

CAN DRUGS CAUSE OSTEOARTHRITIS?

Some medications taken for other diseases can accelerate osteoarthritis. For example, glucocorticoids, or prednisone, is commonly taken for noninfectious inflammatory diseases, slows down articular cartilage replacement and may over time increase the development of osteoarthritis. Strong pain medications that are morphine derivatives (codeine, Darvon, etc.) can mask the pain of osteoarthritis so much that a person can overuse their joints and wear them out faster. It is important to remember that pain has a physiologic function: if a joint produces pain when it is used, it is a signal to use that joint less. A recent study focused on a group of patients with hip osteoarthritis who needed to have a joint replacement in the not-too-distant future. They were randomly prescribed either an anti-inflammatory, aspirin-like drug or an acetaminophen-like drug. Over the next months, the patients were asked about their joint pain, and radiographs of their hips were taken. The patients given the anti-inflammatory drugs had more progression of their hip radiographs and needed to have joint replacements performed in half the time as the group given acetaminophens. It is not known why the subjects in the anti-inflammatory group needed to have the hip replacements sooner; however, there are a few possible explanations. The anti-inflammatory agent might have prevented normal cartilage turnover and repair, and accelerated the joint degeneration; or, more likely, the potent medication decreased joint pain and those subjects were therefore more active. This has led to the suggestion that potent anti-inflammatory medications can lead to the syndrome of "analgesic hip," which can develop if potent pain medication is taken and used continually, thus increasing joint use and leading to accelerated joint degeneration, with a need for joint replacement. A number of studies are now underway to determine if long-term anti-inflammatory use is associated with accelerated progression of knee osteoarthritis. Since analgesics and anti-inflammatory medications are used by millions of Americans every day, the answer to this question is worth knowing.

Another group of medications that may alter joint breakdown in osteoarthritis are the nitrates, including nitroglycerin. Our research group made a preliminary report that use of nitrates over an 8-year period in elderly Caucasian women was associated with a two fold increased risk for developing hip osteoarthritis. Since women who are using nitrates regularly are most likely have heart disease, and chest pain occurs with activity, these women are not very active. Therefore, the reason that nitrates would increase hip osteoarthritis is not immediately clear. However, nitrates are broken down to nitric oxide, which can increase the activity of enzymes that wear down cartilage and at other times increase the proteins that stimulate new bone production. We suspect that the nitric oxide is producing an increase in the enzymes that break down cartilage, and we are further evaluating this finding to determine if nitrate use is associated with both the development and progression of hip and knee osteoarthritis.

WHAT ABOUT WEAK MUSCLES?

Muscles surrounding the joints are important protective shock absorbers. If the muscles around the joint weaken, then the joint receives higher loads. Over time, this can accelerate the degeneration of the joint. Recently, a study of individuals with knee osteoarthritis found that muscle weakness, and *not* knee osteoarthritis, resulted in knee pain. These findings need to be validated in other studies, but it could be that muscle strength might prevent the development or progression of osteoarthritis. Further support for muscle strength affecting osteoarthritis is that individuals who exercise tend to have good muscle strength, and this may prevent joint degeneration in recreational athletes. Also, when subjects develop osteoarthritis, a muscle-strengthening program to improve strength around the joint can reduce pain and may also prevent the progression of the disease. Therefore, muscle strength may play a direct role in the progression of osteoarthritis, especially in weight-bearing joints.

DOES BONE MASS INFLUENCE OSTEOARTHRITIS?

A number of studies have found that high bone mass increases the risk of developing osteoarthritis. In one, Caucasian women with a mean age of 70 had their hands, spines, and hips radiographed, and bone mineral densities of the spine, hip, and heel were obtained. Women with hip osteoarthritis had bone mass of the spine almost 10% higher, and about 5% higher than women without hip osteoarthritis. Similarly, women with knee and hand osteoarthritis had both spine and hip bone mass that was higher than women without knee osteoarthritis. This leads one to hypothesize that high bone mass may predispose someone to developing osteoarthritis through a genetic connection, or that high bone mass is a risk factor for osteoarthritis because individuals with heavy

Table 3: Risk factors for developing osteoarthritis

Increased age
Above normal weight
Female
African-American
Certain collagen genes
Joint injury
"Wear and tear"
Certain occupations associated with kneeling and squatting
Vitamin D deficiency
Medications: corticosteroids, certain anti-inflammatories, nitrates
Muscle weakness
Increased bone mass

bones weigh more than individuals who do not have high bone mass. It is not yet clear what the connection is, but individuals with osteoarthritis do have higher bone mass than individuals who do not have the disease, and there is an inverse relationship between osteoporosis (thin fragile bone) and osteoarthritis.

WHAT ABOUT SMOKING?

Some habits can have an influence upon the development and progression of osteoarthritis. Individuals who smoke cigarettes have a lower risk for developing knee and hip osteoarthritis than individuals who do not smoke, for example. The reason for this is not clear. It may be that these individuals are less active and use their joint less, or it may represent a direct effect of the nicotine on cartilage. Whatever the reason, it is safe to say that a small possible reduction in the risk of osteoarthritis from smoking is outweighed by its risks.

Part II

BONING UP ON THE MUSCULOSKELETAL SYSTEM

Though it be disfigured by many defects, to whom is his own body not dear?

—Palachantra, 1 (5th century A.D.)

In order to have arthritis, there must exist a problem with bones, joints, cartilage, or their supporting structures. Chapters 4 and 5 explore how the normal musculoskeletal system is constructed and articulated. The ways in which the system can be deconstructed and disarticulated, resulting in osteoarthritis, are reviewed in a general sense (Part IV will specify these changes in specific parts of the body). How and why does this happen? Chapter 6 will review the mechanisms by which degenerative joint disease evolves.

4

Bone

A Living Tissue

And he said onto me, Son of man, can these bones live?
—Ezekiel 37:3

Most of us think of bones in the skeletal sense . . . dry, inert, and having only a supporting function. However, bones are full of life. Blood vessels flow through them, and bones are constantly being built or eaten away. This chapter will review the structure of bone as it applies to understanding osteoarthritis.

HOW ARE BONES STRUCTURED?

The human skeleton consists of 212 bones and 100 joints in a continuous living dynamic. Joints are surrounded by bone and cartilage. Bone and cartilage communicate with each other and both change as osteoarthritis develops and progresses. Therefore, an understanding of bone is critical to understanding osteoarthritis.

There are two major types of bone in the body. *Cortical bone* forms the outer envelope of bone around the marrow cavity and makes up 80% of the bone in the body. The other major type is *trabecular* (cancellous) bone, which is spread throughout the bone marrow. It is made up of many small thin trabecular lattices and within these lattices is bone marrow. The trabecular bone sits next to the bone marrow: it has a high surface area, and turns over more rapidly. It is the trabecular bone that changes in response to metabolic and hormonal changes. For example, trabecular bone is lost with estrogen deficiency that occurs when women go through menopause, and when a person takes a steroid medication such as prednisone. Cortical bone, on the other hand, is a very strong compact bone and has a very slow turnover rate. Since cortical bone serves as an outer envelope that surrounds the bone marrow, its slow turnover rate has most likely evolved over years. Cortical bone responds to changes in mechanical stress. If you exercise and strengthen your muscles, cortical bone will thicken to some extent. With aging, cortical bone is lost from both a decrease in activity (which weakens muscles) and decreases in cortical bone.

When bone mass is measured by machines referred to as densitometers, a bone mass measurement is taken that is a composite of both cortical and trabecular bone. The areas in the body that are rich in trabecular bone include the vertebrae of the spine, the femoral neck of the hip, and the distal ends of the long bones. Areas rich in cortical bone include the shafts of all the long bones.

THE LIFE CYCLE OF BONE CELLS:
OSTEOCLASTS AND OSTEOBLASTS

Bone is a living organ and is continually renewing itself. The cycle of bone remodeling starts with *osteoclasts* from the bone marrow attaching to the surface of the bone. The osteoclast digs a resorption pit, and then the cell dies. This is followed by the arrival of an *osteoblast* (or bone forming cell, from the bone marrow) and this cell fills in the resorption pit. The osteoblast has three fates: it can differentiate into an osteocyte and stay inside the mineralized bone matrix and communicate with other cells through thin networks; it may become a lining cell that sits on the surface of the bone; or it can die. Debris from resorbed bone enters the bloodstream, which further breaks it down. The cycle of bone remodeling for the trabecular bone takes four to six months in adults, and for cortical bone it is somewhat longer. It is important to remember that bone is remodeling throughout your body all the time, and nearly 10% of your entire skeleton is remodeled each year. There is no doubt that bone is metabolically a very active tissue.

HOW DOES BONE ADJUST TO
OSTEOARTHRITIC CHANGES?

Since this is a book on osteoarthritis, we want to focus on the bone that surrounds the joints. As shown in Figure 1, bone that surrounds the joints is a combination of both cortical bone and trabecular bone. In osteoarthritis, bone next to the joint (known as *subchondral* bone) thickens and new bone forms at the margins of the joint. On radiographs, the thickening of the subchondral bone is referred to as "subchondral sclerosis" and the new bone formation is referred to as *osteophytes* (bone spurs). New osteophytes grow from the end of the articular cartilage. Though this is in an unusual location, it is histologically bone (that is, its tissue and cellular elements are nearly the same). New bone forming at the ends of the joints is thought to be a result of cartilage deterioration. When the cartilage begins to degenerate, it can no longer be an efffective shock absorber; new bone is believed to form in an attempt to act as the shock absorber that cartilage cannot. It is not clear if the osteophyte is an effective shock absorber, because the joint continues to degenerate, the osteophytes grow larger and, after awhile, the joint completely degenerates, possibly necessitating a joint replacement.

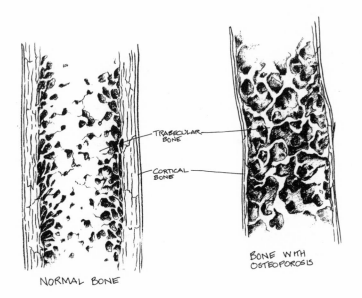

FIG. 1   *Cortical and Trabecular Bone*

As osteophytes are growing out at the margin of the joint, the bone beneath the joint, the subchondral bone, is also thickening. Just as with osteophytes, this is hypothesized to be an additional shock absorber as cartilage degenerates. As the disease progresses, this thickening continues beneath the articular cartilage zone.

In general, individuals with an advanced stage of osteoarthritis have more bone around their joints (and sometimes throughout their bodies) than those individuals without osteoarthritis. While osteoarthritis is a disease that begins with articular cartilage, since the bone sits right next to the cartilage changes also occur in the bone at the beginning of osteoarthritis and as it progresses. Over the years, osteoarthritis experts have debated whether it is a disease of the cartilage or a disease of the bone. Osteoarthritis is clearly a disease that results from cartilage injury, but changes occur in the bone simultaneously. If we are ever to have a treatment to prevent the progression of osteoarthritis, it will most likely need to have effects on both the bone and the cartilage.

DO MENOPAUSE AND HORMONES INFLUENCE BONE METABOLISM?

There are times in one's life that bone is more active than other times. For example, when women start menopause and their estrogen levels decrease, bone turnover increases. Bone resorption by the osteoclasts is faster and more efficient than bone formation, and therefore more bone is lost than is formed for each remodeling cycle. In addition, estrogen deficiency bone loss occurs mostly in the trabecular bone, due to its high turnover rate; since this is the type of bone in the spine, this can result in loss of height and cause compression fractures in the spine. When women go into menopause they often take estrogen or a combination of estrogen and progesterone to prevent this type of bone loss. As long as estrogen is taken, bone remains at its premenopausal mass, but if estrogen is stopped for awhile, the body will quickly increase its bone turnover. Today there are many bone active agents (bisphosphonates, selective estrogen receptor modulators, etc.) available to help prevent estrogen deficient bone loss.

HOW DOES ACTIVITY INFLUENCE BONE METABOLISM?

An example of high turnover bone loss occurs when someone is bedridden. If someone who is active must be restricted to bed for a few months, the body immediately responds to the reduced activity by starting bone remodeling. Since the body senses that it is not as active as it was, it resorbs bone. As bone resorption increases and becomes greater than bone formation, bone loss occurs. When the individual resumes normal activity the bone will again start remodeling, but it will also add more bone than it breaks down because the body needs more bone to be active than it did when the person was bedbound.

SUMMARY

Bones are living organs which are in a constant state of building and breaking down. Structurally, bone can be firm (cortical) or grainy (trabecular), the latter being more influenced by hormonal changes in women. Our body reacts to changes which occur in osteoarthritis by building new bony material in different locations than usual. Menopause and inactivity adversely affect bone metabolism, while hormonal replacement and exercise help rebuild bone.

5

Cartilage and Its Accomplices

The Body's Shock Absorbers

And I kept telling you I ached!
— Anonymous epitaph,
V. Locknar, *Croatian Medical Quotations*

Osteoarthritis is mostly a disease of cartilage. Cartilage is a dense, rubbery or sponge-like material that serves a number of functions in the body. It gives shape and stability of the ear lobe and nose, provides supporting structure for the vocal cords and airways (the trachea and the bronchi within the lung), and makes up material in discs, allowing the spine to provide shock absorption or cushioning. All bones in our skeletons begin as cartilage. As the skeleton matures, cartilage is replaced with hard tissue or bone. Here we will review the structure and function of cartilage in the context of how it influences osteoarthritis.

WHAT IS CARTILAGE MADE UP OF?

There are three types of cartilage in our bodies. *Hyaline cartilage* is the most abundant form, found in the hips, knees, and fingers. *Fibrocartilage* is localized in the discs of the spine, between the vertebrae, and provides shock absorbing ability. *Elastic cartilage* is found around the ear.

Hyaline cartilage in our joints is referred to in this book as *articular cartilage*. It is whitish in color, extremely tough, and elastic. These physical properties of cartilage arise from its components. The major con-

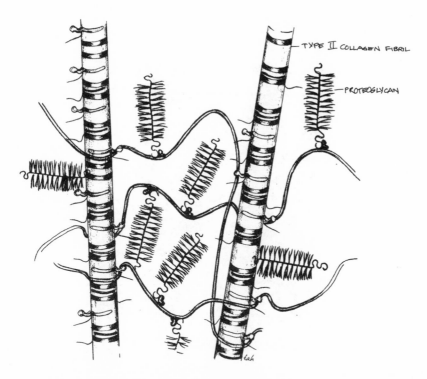

FIG. 2   *The Organization of Articular Cartilage Matrix*

stituents of cartilage are water (nearly 65%), *proteoglycans*, and *collagens*. The proteoglycans (shown in Figure 2) have a protein core with sugars that are attached as side chains called *glucosaminoglycans*, made up mostly of chondroitin sulfate and keratin sulfate. These proteoglycans form aggregates with hyaluronic acid (another glucosaminoglycan) and a link protein, which together contribute to the strength of cartilage. The collagens also are important to the structural integrity and function of cartilage. Type II collagen is the principal type found in hyaline cartilage, but small amounts of other collagens are also found.

Cells embedded through out the cartilage are called *chondrocytes*. These are very interesting cells; because there is no blood supply in cartilage, they must receive all of their nutrients by diffusion of materials. These cells are among the most metabolically active in the body. Chondrocytes are responsible for synthesizing proteins that make up cartilage, as well as in the enzymes that break down cartilage in both normal turnover and disease states such as osteoarthritis. (See Figure 3.)

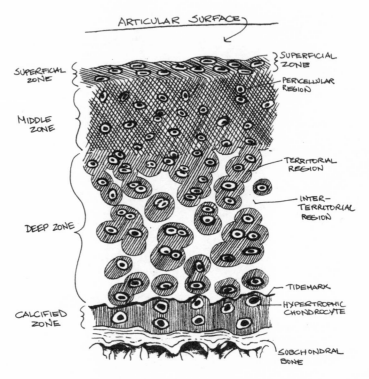

FIG. 3   *The Articular Surface of Cartilage*

The chondrocyte produces a number of enzymes that we refer to as *metalloproteinases*, which break down cartilage under normal and abnormal conditions. For example, *stromelysin* breaks down proteoglycans, *collagenase* breaks down the collagen, and gelatinase also breaks down collagen. Another type of metalloproteinase enzymes, *tissue inhibitors of metalloproteinases* (TIMPs) are naturally occurring small proteins which inhibit metalloproteinases so that they do not break down too much cartilage. Under normal conditions these enzymes are found in very low concentrations in cartilage with normal levels of their inhibitors, the TIMPs. In abnormal conditions, however, the levels of these enzymes increases and TIMPs decrease. They break down cartilage faster than the chondrocyte can make new cartilage, resulting in a loss of cartilage.

HOW DOES CARTILAGE FUNCTION?

The major function of articular cartilage is to provide shock absorption for bones in a joint. Proteoglycans act as shock absorbers; they take in

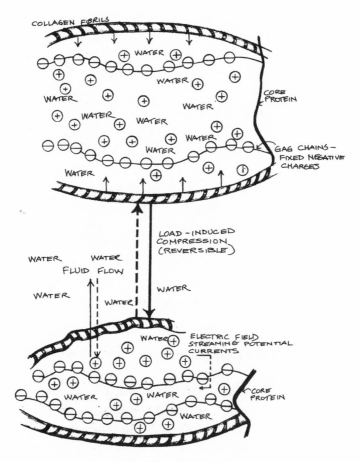

FIG. 4   *How Cartilage Acts as a Shock Absorber*

water when you take weight off your joints and push water out when you put weight on a joint like the knee. Like a sponge, this provides important buffering protection. The other important function of cartilage is as a lubricant. Like oil, its slipperiness allows joint surfaces to slide back and forth with very little friction. While proteoglycans are the shock absorbers of the joint, collagen is a strong fibrous protein providing the main framework for cartilage. Collagen in the joint forms a structure like a net, to hold the proteoglycans and water. This net provides cartilage with its shape and tensile strength. Since collagen is a very stiff material, proteoglycans spread throughout the collagen net are flexible, and give cartilage its ability to stretch with movement.

Cartilage is an amazing physiologically active material. The chondrocyte cells, buried within the cartilage matrix, synthesize materials that build the matrix up and enzymes that break it down. For example, when cartilage is functioning well, it has the properties necessary for us to walk. When walking, we put heavy loads on our legs. Cartilage responds to this load by releasing fluid stored in its matrix. Releasing the fluid cushions the load on the ends of the bones and keeps them from rubbing against each other. When the load is shifted to the other leg, cartilage quickly reabsorbs the fluid it expelled, preparing the joints of the lower leg for the next step. In non-weight-bearing joints such as the shoulders, elbows, wrists, and fingers, the slippery nature of the cartilage allows for continuous and smooth movements. (See Figure 4.)

Cartilage was designed to last a lifetime. Under normal conditions, just like bone, it continuously turns its tissue or matrix over. Chondrocytes produce enough new cartilage matrix to replace worn out collagen and proteoglycan components. Many factors, however—some that we know and some that we do not—destroy or interfere with this delicate balance. Over time this leads to osteoarthritis.

CARTILAGE AND ASSOCIATED TISSUES

Ligaments are tough structures made of collagen, which surround our joints and connect bone. These structures keep the joint aligned. Medial and lateral ligaments surround the knee, and the anterior cruciate ligaments connect the femur and the tibia inside the knee joint. Weakness or loosening of ligaments from injuries or degeneration results in misalignment of joints, which accelerates their degeneration. Within the knee there is a dense layer of cartilage known as *menisci*. These structures function as strong shock absorbers. Resembling white discs, menisci are frequently torn in athletic injuries, and also with age. Often menisci fray and degenerate in osteoarthritis.

Muscles are critical to joint health. By surrounding joints, muscles help absorb the shock transmitted through use, and also keep joints in alignment. When a knee begins to become osteoarthritic, for example, muscles around it weaken and pain occurs. Strong muscles around joints can prevent pain. It is possible that good muscle strength can slow the progression of osteoarthritis in weight-bearing joints.

Table 4: The structure of cartilage

TYPES OF CARTILAGE

Hyaline (articular) cartilage (its degeneration causes osteoarthritis)
    Contains chondrocytes which make all components of hyaline cartilage and
    metalloproteinase enzymes that degrade cartilage.
Fibrocartilage
Elastic cartilage

COMPONENTS OF HYALINE CARTILAGE

Water
Proteoglycans (broken down by stromolysin)
    Contains glucosaminoglycans: chondroitin sulfate, keratin sulfate, hyaluronic
    acid and others
Collagens
    Type II is the most important; broken down by collagenase and gelatinase

SUMMARY

Osteoarthritis is a disease of cartilage. Acting as a shock absorber and
lubricant, cartilage protects bones from rubbing against each other and
promotes friction-free movement. Though cartilage is avascular, cartilage cells are very metabolically active. Working with bones, muscles,
tendons, ligaments, and other supporting structures, cartilage responds
to our daily joint loading and maintains a high level of mobility and
functioning throughout life.

6

What Causes Osteoarthritis?

Clear and precise definitions of disease . . . are of more conse-
quence than they are generally imagined to be; untrue or im-
perfect ones occasion false ideas, and false ideas are generally
followed by erroneous practice.

—Percival Pott (1765),
A Treatise on Fistula in Ano

What sets in motion the sequence of events that leads to osteoarthritis? We already know that certain populations, such as women and the elderly, are predisposed, and that a variety of environmental factors such as occupation, weight, exercise, and trauma further increase one's risk of developing osteoarthritis. But what actually initiates the process, and how does the disease progress?

THE INITIATING EVENT

Many theories have been proposed to explain the degeneration of the articular cartilage in osteoarthritis. The initiating event is most likely from a mechanical stress that leads to altered chondrocyte activities. The chondrocyte increases its production of enzymes, referred to as a group as *metalloproteinase* enzymes. These enzymes break down the cartilage matrix, and the cartilage loses some of its unique functional properties.

Certain events can lead to abnormal mechanical stress with a biologic response, initiating the cascade of cartilage breakdown, joint pain, and osteoarthritis. Examples include:

· a sports injury damaging the meniscus of the knee
· a broken bone which places stresses to the joints and cartilage as it heals
· a person with a genetically abnormal type II collagen protein which prematurely breaks down
· an overweight individual who sends increased forces to a joint
· a factory worker that bends and lifts objects often during the day

THE PERPETUATING CASCADE

Whatever the initiating event, osteoarthritis results from an abnormal mechanical force that sends proteins called *cytokines* to signal the chondrocyte to produce the enzymes which start the process of cartilage breakdown. Over time, this can lead to osteoarthritis. Some of these cytokines include interleukin-1 (IL-1), tumor necrosis factor (TNF), and interleukin-6 (IL-6).

In early osteoarthritis, mechanical stresses are just the beginning. The chondrocyte tries to respond by dividing into more chondrocytes or cloning and forming clusters within the cartilage. These chondrocytes produce increased amounts of cytokines (IL-1, IL-6, TNF), growth factors, metalloproteinase enzymes, and many other enzymes. Cytokines signal the chondrocyte to produce metalloproteinase enzymes that degrade proteoglycan and collagen and block the synthesis of new cartilage matrix proteins. Cytokines also decrease the production of natural tissue inhibitors of the metalloproteinase enzymes (TIMPs) so that there is no way to stop these enzymes from breaking down cartilage. The imbalance between the production of metalloproteinase enzymes and the TIMPs tips the scale in favor of increased cartilage breakdown and the development of osteoarthritis.

Once the osteoarthritis process is started in cartilage, it progresses. Over time, cartilage architecture changes and the mechanical forces to the joint are further increased. This leads to more stress on the joint, and more production of cartilage-degrading enzymes. The process of joint destruction in osteoarthritis often becomes a self-perpetuating process.

Some doctors think that crystals released into the joints, and cause pain and joint swelling can also cause osteoarthritis. This is probably not true. During the destructive phase of osteoarthritis, crystals are shed from cartilage into joint fluid. These crystals are usually made of calcium phosphate or hydroxyapatite. Once these crystals are released they set off a very painful inflammatory response and the joint swells up and becomes red. The swelling usually lasts a few days. Exactly why some people with osteoarthritis have crystal shedding and inflammation and others do not is not known. It may simply be part of the cartilage degeneration process in some people and can be referred to as pseudo-gout, calcium pyrophosphate deposition disease (CPPD), or a gout-like attack. This will be discussed in more detail in chapter 9.

SUMMARY

Some individuals posess predisposing factors for osteoarthritis, which in combination with environmental factors or trauma place mechanical stress on joints. The chondrocyte cells respond by dividing and releasing cytokines and enzymes. These chemicals work to both protect and damage cartilage, but the balance tips in favor of cartilage breakdown. Ultimately this leads to osteoarthritis.

Part III

HOW DOES A DOCTOR EVALUATE OSTEOARTHRITIS?

The whole body becomes painful . . . the pain rages especially about the joints, so that indeed neither the foot nor the hand, nor the finger can be moved . . . without pain or outcry . . . Although the arthritis is in a certain part, this rheumatism it-self is in the entire body.

—Guillaume de Baillou (Ballonius),
Opera Medica Omnia (1736)

When arthritis pain begins, most people hurt enough to discuss it with their doctor. How can the doctor tell what kind of arthritis it is? What should be done at a physical examination? Are X-rays of afflicted areas useful? Can blood testing, scans, electrical studies, or biopsies tell us anything? Once your doctor relates that it is, indeed, osteoarthritis, how can he or she be sure it's not some other type of musculoskeletal condition? Chapters 7 through 10 will address these issues.

7

What Happens at a Musculoskeletal Examination?

Doctors think a lot of patients are cured who have simply quit in disgust.

—Don Herold

Something is not right. It's not that you don't feel well, but something different is going on. It could be that you are newly stiff, achy, or have noticed a deformity on your hand. What needs to be done? Who should you see? This chapter will guide you to a physician who can evaluate musculoskeletal complaints, initiate a diagnostic workup, and recommend treatment.

I HURT. WHO SHOULD I SEE TO EVALUATE MY COMPLAINT?

There is a seemingly bewildering array of musculoskeletal specialists. Some are physicians; others are not. (Chapter 22 reviews the responsibilities of these practitioners.) However, for all practical purposes, a primary care physician should be your starting point. These doctors are general practitioners, family practitioners, or internal medicine specialists, depending on the amount of training and expertise they have. For patients who have Health Maintenance Organization (HMO) or Point of Service (POS) plans, there is often no choice. These physicians serve a "gatekeeper" function, and evaluate initial complaints. If your case is more complicated and your symptoms cannot be easily relieved, these

doctors may refer you to a musculoskeletal specialist. If they don't, take
charge and never be afraid to ask for a referral. After all, it's your body!

WHAT HAPPENS AT A PRIMARY CARE DOCTOR'S MUSCULOSKELETAL EVALUATION?

Primary care physicians have a wide variety of expertise in evaluating
joint and muscle complaints. In some family practice programs, rheumatology rotations are limited to two weeks out of three years of training.
On the other hand, at least 2,000 of the 5,000 rheumatologists in the
United States practice primary care internal medicine in addition to
consultative rheumatology.

The chief complaints of an osteoarthritis patient are usually fairly consistent and focused. These include pain, stiffness, swelling, weakness, deformity, fatigue, or decreased range of motion. Complaints that are subjective
are known as *symptoms*, and those, found during a physical examination
are termed *signs*. The principal constellation of symptoms and signs of osteoarthritis are listed in Table 5, at the end of this chapter. At your musculoskeletal examination, the primary care doctor will probably ask what
your complaints are (symptoms), take a medical history, perform a physical examination (looking for signs), and obtain blood testing, imaging
studies (X-rays or scans), and, if needed, other diagnostic investigations.
The primary care doctor will then decide whether to treat your complaints,
start therapy, or refer you to a specialist or allied health professional.

OSTEOARTHRITIS SYMPTOMS

Stiffness is commonly present in osteoarthritis. It usually occurs in the
morning, and joints feel gel-like or "stuck." The stiffness usually lasts for
10–30 minutes and disappears upon limbering up. Gelling occcurs after periods of inactivity, such as sleeping. It is a discomfort or restriction perceived as one attempts their first easy movements in the morning. Stiffness
usually occurs in areas involved by arthritis, and improves with activity,
moist heat, or a hot shower or bath. Stiffness that lasts longer than an hour
should warrant your doctor to perform tests looking for other rheumatic
conditions such as rheumatoid arthritis, ankylosing spondylitis, polymyalgia rheumatica, or systemic lupus. Patients who complain of stiffness in the
afternoon or evening often have a form of soft tissue rheumatism known as

fibromyalgia. What causes stiffness? Nobody knows, but it is thought to be due to chemical interactions within a joint that is not used for several hours.

Fatigue is a subjective sensation of loss of stamina or decreased endurance, which makes it difficult to carry out normal daily activities. Usually, osteoarthritis is not associated with fatigue. However, when osteoarthritis is part of an inflammatory process, such as a herniated disc, pseudo-gout with swollen joints, or inflammatory osteoarthritis, fatigue can be present but is mild and not overwhelming. Since osteoarthritis patients may have additional musculoskeletal or medical conditions, the presence of fatigue should warrant a search for the following causes: metabolic (e.g, thyroid, diabetes, malnutrition); infectious (such as a virus); inflammatory (rheumatoid arthritis, lupus); mechanical or internal derangement (a fracture or torn ligament); allergic; psychiatric (depression, substance abuse); hematologic (such as anemia); fibromatous; hormonal (e.g., menopause); or neurologic (for example multiple sclerosis or Parkinson's).

Sometimes, in addition to feeling tired, one can sense *weakness*. Although weakness can be a subjective sensation, the objective loss of motor power or muscular strength occurs with advanced osteoarthritis. Destructive joint changes produce muscle weakness, which makes it hard to walk, work, or perform daily activities. These changes are usually localized. *However*, if the weakness is generalized, all the causes of fatigue (as noted in the above paragraph) need to be considered in addition to muscle diseases and drug reactions. Sometimes, the sense of weakness reflects a tendency for the knees to buckle, or lock. This is caused by loose bodies or floating cartilage fragments within a joint.

> Nikki recently turned 48. For the first time, she began feeling stiffness in her fingers in the morning with minimal aching. A hot shower relieved the discomfort, but over the following months she noticed a knobby appearance in her small finger joints. Dr. Wu assured Nikki that she was developing a mild, early form of osteoarthritis. Nikki's mother related that the same thing happened to her at that age, and other than taking an occasional Advil, the stiffness and pain was never severe enough to do anything about it.

Joint pain, especially manifested by aching, is the most common symptom of osteoarthritis that sends patients to a doctor. Pain is subjective, complex, and difficult to explain. Patients in pain usually look and behave normally. Mood, personality, emotional status, and past conditioning influence one's reaction to pain and pain thresholds. Since many disorders are associated with joint pain, your doctor might wish to take a more detailed history: Which joints are involved? Distribution is important, since rheumatoid arthritis tends to first involve multiple small joints of the hands and feet, while ankylosing spondylitis starts in the low back. Does the pain involve areas other than joints, such as the muscles or soft tissues? Is the pain localized or deep, and what is its character? Is it crampy, persistent, intermittent, boring, or a shooting pain, as experience with nerve injuries? Is there numbness, tingling, or burning associated with it? Is it severe or intense? When did it start? Was there an injury? What activities make the pain better or worse? Is it getting better or worse? How long has the discomfort been present and what have you done for it? What can't you do as a result of this? Has your lifestyle changed in any way? Are there associated manifestations with the pain such as a rash, fever, feeling of lightheadedness, or headache?

Osteoarthritis pain is usually localized to the involved joint, and is not associated with systemic symptoms. The onset of osteoarthritis in a joint can be accelerated by an injury, repetitive motions at work or recreationally, or may be secondary to an inflammatory condition such as gout. If pain is due to inflammation, it usually responds to anti-inflammatory drug regimens. However, if the pain is due to deformity or an internal derangement, then analgesic medications, physical therapy measures, local injections, and perhaps surgery could be indicated.

HOW DOES A PRIMARY CARE DOCTOR APPROACH A MUSCULOSKELETAL EXAMINATION?

The most common mistake doctors make is to box themselves into a mind-set. For example, if a lupus patient sees a dermatologist for their rash but neglects to tell him or her about their swollen knee, the lupus will never get better. Similarly, when a busy primary care doctor sees you as the thirtieth patient of the day at 4:30 PM and you both are tired, resist temptation to "not bother the doctor" with your problems. If you are complaining of hand pain, make sure that your doctor also asks you if anything else hurts. Bring a list of problems with you. Osteoarthritis is frequently *monoarticular*, affecting one joint at a time. *Polyarthritis*, or pain in multiple joints, is often due to inflammatory processes such as rheumatoid arthritis and warrants a completely different approach.

Based upon the nature of your complaints, your primary care doctor may wish to perform a physical examination. This usually precedes the joint examination. Frequently, the doctor or an assistant will take your vital signs (height, weight, temperature, pulse, and blood pressure). The physical examination may include listening to your heart or lungs, feeling your abdomen, and performing a neurologic evaluation. In the latter, pulses, reflexes, and responses to various maneuvers are evaluated.

The thorough primary care doctor will focus upon those joints which are involved. The joint is first viewed or inspected for swelling, color changes, or deformity. It is then palpated for tenderness, warmth, and degree of swelling. A range of motion examination follows as the joint is flexed, extended, abducted (moved out), adducted (moved inward), or rotated. Abnormal sounds can sometimes be heard when the joints are put through a range of motion. Limitation of joint movement is carefully noted. Since arthritic complaints frequently overlap with neurologic symptoms or poor circulation, many doctors also examine the patient's peripheral pulses, reflexes and muscular strength. (Specific maneuvers germane to regions of the body are reviewed in Chapters 11–13.)

When some of us are in our 40s, we begin to notice a knobbiness in our knuckles and small finger joints. Our mothers may have experienced the same thing. This hereditary form of osteoarthritis, known as Hebreden's nodes, is the most common presenting *deformity* seen with the disorder. (The pathophysiologic process by which this occurs has been reviewed in Chapter 6.) While usually not painful, it can be associated with some discomfort, especially during the first year that it appears. Joint-space narrowing, osteophytes, malalignment of joints, and the degradation of cartilage all lead to deformities. *Color changes* in the skin are not associated with osteoarthritis, but could indicate an autoimmune, autonomic, or vascular problem—an infection such as cellulitis or crystals in the joint, as seen in gout. *Joint swelling* can be a subjective sensation of fullness or objective evidence for fluid within a joint capsule. Patients with congestive heart failure, circulation problems, or lupus in their kidney can have swollen ankles without any arthritis, due to fluid retention. Individuals with fibromyalgia complain of retaining fluid in their tissues and commonly ask for diuretics (water pills), even though there is no visible swelling. Fluid in a joint capsule may or may not be painful. In osteoarthritis, patients are frequently unaware of small amounts of fluid and the area is not tender. Arthritis specialists have evolved techniques of "balloting" or maneuvering a joint to estimate how much fluid is present and whether the fluid is within the joint or one of its adjacent bursae (the sacs cushioning the joint). Painful swelling usually implies that an inflammatory process is ongo-

Table 5: Symptoms and signs associated with osteoarthritis

Symptoms (Patient complaints)	Signs (Physical findings)
Pain	Discomfort or abnormality with motion
Stiffness	Limitation in stamina or endurance
Swelling	Color changes
Achy muscles or joints	Swelling
Fatigue	Warmth or tenderness to touch
Weakness	Crepitation
Deformity	Abnormal posture or gait

ing. In osteoarthritis this can be due to a secondary inflammatory condition such as gout or rheumatoid arthritis, or total loss of cartilage in a destroyed joint where bone is grating on bone and joint fluid can accumulate. *Joint tenderness* in osteoarthritis is also associated with internal derangements such as a bursitis, tendonitis, a torn meniscus or a torn ligament. If the skin or muscle is also tender away from the joint, a syndrome known as fibromyalgia should be suspected. *Crepitation* can produce cracking sounds when tendons or ligaments slip over body surfaces in motion, as well as being an audible grating or crunching sensation from roughened cartilaginous surfaces. Finally, your doctor might move the joint in all possible directions to look for limitations in its *range of motion*. This allows one to ascertain the consequences of deformity, locking, joint effusions, or contractures. Are there differences in limb length or digit length? Do the muscles look wasted or atrophied? When walking, are there abnormalities in posture or gait?

MY DOCTOR HAS LISTENED TO ME AND EXAMINED WHERE I HURT. WHAT NOW?

Once a practitioner has heard your complaint, asked all the questions necessary to limit its scope, and determined how long you've had the problem and what you have done about it, he or she can stop at this juncture and make a treatment recommendation, refer you to a specialist, or initiate diagnostic testing. Most primary care doctors have ready access to an X-ray machine and clinical laboratory and are skilled at interpreting their results. Occasionally, they may request specialized scans, vascular reports, or electrical studies. (These are reviewed in the next chapter.) And don't worry—there are plenty of effective therapies that we will discuss later.

8

How Is Osteoarthritis Diagnosed?

Blood will tell, but it often tells too much.

—Don Marquis (1878–1937)

"My doctor says I have osteoarthritis," a patient tells her friend. "How do you know?" is the reply. Since there are no diagnostic blood or urine tests for the disorder, the label osteoarthritis all too often seems to be one of exclusion, once other possibilities have been considered. In fact, osteoarthritis is so prevalent that it often coexists with many other musculoskeletal disorders. So how can we tell you have osteoarthritis?

BLOOD TESTS

There are a wide variety of arthritis blood tests physicians can order. These determinations can suggest if something is wrong with the musculoskeletal system. Let's start with the blood evaluations that primary care physicians routinely order at a check-up. A low red blood count, or anemia, might indicate a chronic inflammatory process such as rheumatoid arthritis or lupus. Low white blood cell or platelet counts are also seen in patients with autoimmune disorders. From the results of a blood chemistry panel, doctors consider that low thyroid levels can produce joint pains; an elevated alkaline phosphatase can be associated with bone inflammation, Paget's disease, or tumors; a high uric acid is related to gout, and an elevated creatine phosphokinase (CPK) can mean muscle inflammation. Inflammatory arthritis (gout, rheumatoid arthritis, lupus, ankylosing spondylitis) and infections result in elevations in the sedimentation rate or C-reactive protein (CRP). Protein or blood in the urine are commonly found in autoimmune disorders. However, even if you have an inflammatory form of osteoarthritis, all of these tests are usually normal.

Primary care doctors often order some relatively inexpensive, readily available serologic tests to look for different antibodies, proteins, or markers in the blood. These include an antinuclear antibody (ANA), rheumatoid factor, and an HLA-B27. If they are negative, it goes against the diagnosis of rheumatoid arthritis, lupus, ankylosing spondylitis, or a reactive arthritis. Arthritis blood testing is summarized in Table 6.

Table 6: Arthritis blood tests

Blood Test	Clinical Use
Sedimentation rate	Elevated with inflammation
C-Reactive protein (CRP)	Elevated with inflammation and infection
White blood cell count	Increased with inflammation, infection, or stress
Platelet counts	Platelets clot blood; low in autoimmune disease, high in infection and some types of inflammation
Hemoglobin	If low, patient is anemic; low in autoimmune disease
Uric Acid	Increased levels associated with gout
Alkaline phosphatase	Increased with bone activity, inflammation, tumors
Creatine phosphokinase (CPK)	A muscle enzyme increased with inflammation
Antinuclear antibody (ANA)	Present in autoimmune disease, especially lupus
Rheumatoid factor (RA)	Present in 70% of patients with rheumatoid arthritis
HLA–B27	Positive in ankylosing spondylitis, reactive arthritis

So, is there any point in doing blood testing for osteoarthritis patients? The answer is yes. Other considerations need to be ruled out if the diagnosis is not obvious. Once osteoarthritis is diagnosed and treatment is initiated, blood may need to be drawn several times a year to monitor medication.

I HAVE FLUID IN MY KNEE. DOES LOOKING AT FLUID UNDER THE MICROSCOPE HELP?

The *synovium*, or lining of the joint, makes a yellowish liquid which lubricates the joint capsule. When fluid accumulates, your doctor may wish to remove it for diagnostic and/or therapeutic purposes. Diagnostically, joint fluid is cultured to look for infection, and analyzed for crystals (as seen in gout and pseudo-gout), protein (increased with inflammation), and cell count. The cell count measures the number of white blood cells in the fluid per cubic millimeter. Patients with osteoarthritis or internal derangements (e.g., a torn meniscus) usually have cell counts in the 200–500 range. As a comparison, those with rheumatoid arthritis or lupus average 10,000–50,000 cells, gout averages 50,000–100,000, and those with septic arthritis have counts in the range of 100,000. Therefore, a synovial fluid analysis can be an important diagnostic tool for musculoskeletal specialists.

CAN AN X-RAY HELP MAKE THE DIAGNOSIS?

X-rays create an image of bone, soft tissues, and calcium on a negative photographic plate. The changes in bone and cartilage that occur with osteoarthritis (reviewed in chapters 4–6) are usually easy to visualize on an X-ray. These are shown in Figure 5 and include:

- Joint space narrowing, due to loss of articular cartilage. It is usually asymmetrical.
- Bony proliferation due to osteophytes or bone spurs
- Thickened bone beneath articular cartilage, known as *subchondral sclerosis*
- "Mouse bites," or bone erosions in the far knuckle joints of the hands, indicative of inflammatory osteoarthritis; erosions seen

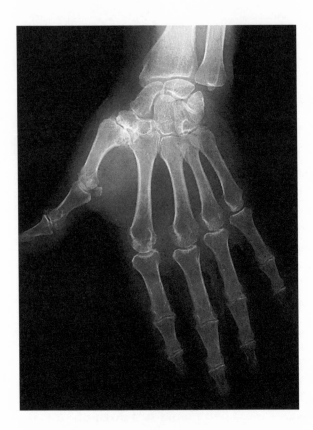

FIG. 5   *(upside down) X-ray of an osteoarthritic hand*

elsewhere suggest rheumatoid arthritis, psoriatic arthritis, gout or a reactive arthritis.

Not everybody with an X-ray showing changes consistent with osteoarthritis has pain or any symptoms. In fact, most do not. Pain results from a variety of factors (discussed in chapter 24). Nevertheless, if pain is present, an X-ray of the involved joint can remove from consideration other forms of arthritis and appropriately direct your doctor's management of the disorder.

Sometimes, contrasts or dyes are used along with plain X-rays to better define structures. In a joint this is called an *arthrogram* and in the spine a *myelogram*. In view of the expense and greater radiation exposure of these procedures, their use has dramatically declined and they are now employed for special circumstances since magnetic resonance imaging (MRI) and computed tomographic (CT) scanning are, in most cases, equally revealing.

MY DOCTOR SAYS AN X-RAY IS NOT GOOD ENOUGH.
WHAT OTHER IMAGING TESTS MIGHT BE ORDERED?

Imaging can evaluate structures in two ways: anatomically and physiologically. The first tells us about the contents of a structure, the latter delineates its function. In addition to a plain X-ray, musculoskeletal specialists may use three additional methods for looking at structures: an ultrasound, CT scan, or MRI scan. When are these procedures indicated? *Ultrasounds* use sound waves to evaluate soft tissue structures. Using no radiation or dyes, the ultrasound is a painless procedure. It can measure cysts, bursae, and masses under the skin, and can evaluate sarcomas, tumors, and measure joint fluid. *CT scans* are highly specialized X-rays, which emit moderate amounts of radiation. CT scans are often the best way to look at bony structures and have excellent resolution to differentiate bone from soft tissues. They can diagnose herniated discs in the back, narrowing of the spinal canal (spinal stenosis), and assess bone mineralization. *MRI scans* use magnets to create images and are free of radiation. Of particular value for herniated discs, spinal stenosis, torn menisci, stress fractures, tumors, and dead bone (avascular necrosis or osteonecrosis), use of the MRI has greatly increased. A modified X-ray, known as *dual X-ray absoptiometry* (DXA), has become the preferred method for evaluating bone mineralization and diagnosing osteoporosis.

Activity within a joint can be discerned by several dynamic imaging techniques. They range from a *bone scan*, where inflamed joints or recently fractured bones "light up" when a special contrast agent known as technetium is injected; *gallium scans*, which identify areas of infections; and single photon emission computed tomography (SPECT), where facet joints of the back can be optimally visualized.

ARE THERE ANY OTHER DIAGNOSTIC STUDIES
MY DOCTOR MIGHT ORDER?

An electrical survey known as an *electromyogram* (EMG) with *nerve conduction velocities* (NCVs) is sometimes ordered for osteoarthritis patients. Essentially an electrocardiogram of the muscles and nerves, electrical impulses captured on tracings can provide your doctor with information about damage produced by bone spurs. For example, bone spurs frequently touch nerves emanating from the back to the legs or from the neck to the arms. An EMG with NCV can tell us whether this is coming from a herniated disc, if it is acute or chronic, whether or not the nerve is damaged, if it is reinnervating, or growing back. Sometimes, a patient with leg pain has osteoarthritis changes on X-ray but the EMG/NCV suggests that the discomfort has nothing to do with the abnormal X-ray. An electrical study may suggest that a musculoskeletal problem could be due to anything from a thyroid disorder, an inflamed muscle, or lead poisoning.

SUMMARY

In addition to listening to your complaints, taking a history, and performing a physical examination, before initiating treatment a doctor may feel the need to acquire additional information. This might include obtaining blood tests, urine tests, X-rays, specialized scans or imaging procedures, or electrical studies. The primary care doctor may then suggest a combination of therapies, initiate treatment, or refer you to a musculoskeletal specialist.

9

The Many Faces of Osteoarthritis

Specialized Forms

I, that am curtail'd of this fair proportion,
Cheated of feature by dissembling nature
Deform'd, unfinish'd, sent before my time
—William Shakespeare (1592), *Richard III*

Although most people view osteoarthritis as simply "arthritis," in reality there are many different types of this misunderstood disorder. As noted in chapter 1, 85–90% of osteoarthritis is known as "generalized" or "primary." In chapters 11–13, we cover specific forms of generalized, primary osteoarthritis, which have unique or special characteristics when they appear in certain parts of the body. Examples of this adaptation to differing anatomic regions include Hebreden's nodes in the small joints of the hand, chondromalacia patellae in the kneecap, spinal stenosis (narrowing of the spinal canal) or herniated discs in the back, and inflammatory or erosive osteoarthritis in the hand. Occasionally, classic osteoarthritis can be accelerated as a consequence of overuse syndromes and "wear and tear," as in a baseball pitcher's shoulder or a basketball player's knee. Trauma clearly brings on primary-appearing osteoarthritis to the area of injury or overuse earlier than it would appear otherwise. Broken bones during childhood often lead to osteoarthritic joints in later years.

Ten to 15% of osteroarthritis derives from conditions that seemingly have little relation with it. For example, what does diabetes have to do with osteoarthritis? This chapter reviews the secondary conditions and associations which result in specialized forms of osteoarthritis.

53

COULD THERE BE A GEOGRAPHIC ROLE
IN OSTEOARTHRITIS?

Endemic osteoarthritis is found in confined geographic areas associated with noninflammatory joint diseases. There are two well-documented examples of endemic osteoarthritis. At least two million persons in Northern China, North Korea, and eastern Siberia have *Kashin-Beck disease*. Thought to derive from selenium deficiency, a fungal toxin in grain, or fulvic acid contamination in water, the processing of type II procollagen to mature type II collagen is inhibited and this leads to developmental abnormalities. It first appears in childhood and leads to profound deformities.

In the northern Zululand region of South Africa, communities with early onset of osteoarthritis (especially of the hip) have been described where X-rays show little eburnation. This suggests that the development of dysplastic spondyloepiphyseal (spinal growth plates) may be causative. This condition is known as *Mseleni joint disease.*

HOW OSTEOARTHRITIS INTERRELATES WITH
METABOLIC DISORDERS AND HORMONES

Crystal induced arthridites and chrondrocalcinosis (gout and pseudo-gout)

> Linda has what she thought to be mild osteoarthritis of her knees. The occasional pain responded to Advil. This time, it was different. Over a period of hours, her right knee swelled up. Having a warm and painful "balloon" in her knee was a new experience. Linda called her internist who sent her to a rheumatologist. Dr. Grange drained the knee, looked at the fluid under a microscope with a special "polarizing" lens and saw calcium pyrophosphate crystals. X-rays of the knee demonstrated crystals spread throughout the articular cartilage joint space (chondrocalcinosis), with medial joint space narrowing consistent with mild osteoarthritis. The joint was injected with a corticosteroid and local anesthetic combination. Linda was prescribed a high dose of Naprosyn for one week and was back to normal a few days later.

Three million Americans have some form of arthritis produced by crystals. When uric acid, cholesterol, basic calcium phosphate, or calcium

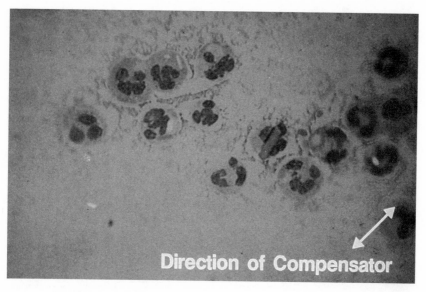

Direction of Compensator

FIG. 6   *Pseudo-gout crystals*

pyrophosphate crystallizes in joints, they can produce severe pain and inflammation. Though over 20 crystal related conditions are associated with joint pain, gout (uric acid crystals) or pseudo-gout (calcium pryophosphate crystals) induce 95% of all cases. Since these are inflammatory arthritic types of conditions, what does this have to do with osteoarthritis? In gout, inflammation of the joint precedes the development of osteoarthritis. In other words, chronic changes in the joint due to repeated inflammatory attacks alter the architecture of the joint in a way that the onset of osteoarthritis is accelerated. Gout usually occurs in only one to two joints at a time and feels likes a "hot poker" pain. Like pseudo-gout, crystal-induced gouty arthritis is a limited process that generally resolves without treatment over a two-week period. These crystals are illustrated in Figure 6. Most doctors manage acute gout with nonsteroidal anti-inflammatory drugs, local injection into the joints with a corticosteroid preparation, and sometimes an anti-inflammatory agent known as *colchicine.*

Pseudo-gout, on the other hand, is usually caused by osteoarthritis. "Crumbs" of cartilage deposited into the joint in osteoarthritis concurrently release basic calcium phosphate and pyrophosphate (and occasionally calcium hydroxyapatite), which form crystals and produce a

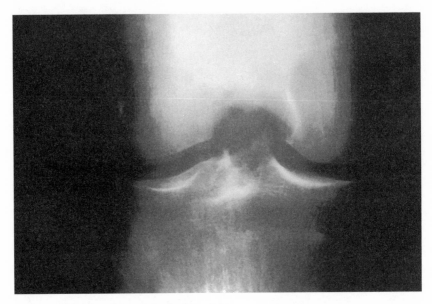

FIG. 7   *Chondrocalcinosis in the knee joint*

secondary inflammatory arthropathy. Another predisposing factor towards pseudo-gout is the finding of *chondrocalcinosis*. This can be diagnosed when calcium deposits are seen in cartilage on an X-ray (Figure
7). This finding is usually associated with the aging process and is
prominently found in the knee. Most patients with chondrocalcinosis
have no symptoms, but when their knee swells up and is painful, we almost always find calcium pyrophosphate crystals. Pseudo-gout is not as
painful as gout, which is characterized by sudden onset of pain in a
lower extremity joint (95% of the time, especially in the big toe).

Pseudo-gout has a less sudden onset than gout, is less inflammatory,
and is frequently found in larger joints (especially the knee). Pseudo-
gout knees may contain large amounts of joint fluid, which respond to
nonsteroidal anti-inflammatory drugs and local corticosteroid injection
with drainage of joint fluid.

Metabolic osteoarthritis: disorders of copper, iron, calcium, and beyond

In chemical parlance, copper, iron, and calcium have a double positive
charge (++). For reasons that are not clear, radiographic chondrocalci-

nosis is found prematurely in patients with disorders of divalent cations (Ca++, Fe++, Cu++), which in turn is associated with osteoarthritis.

Wilson's disease is an inherited disorder characterized by excessive retention of copper, which can produce eye, kidney, and brain changes, as well as liver failure. Patients have mild, premature osteoarthritis in their hands, wrists, knees, and spine. Articular cartilage may contain copper deposits. The disorder is diagnosed by checking a serum ceruloplasmin level; D-penicillamine is the treatment of choice.

In *hemochromatosis*, excessive body iron stores and deposition of an irritating by-product of iron known as *hemosiderin* can produce joint changes as well as liver, heart, and pancreatic failure. Osteoarthritic changes are found in patients as young as 25, especially in the near knuckles of the hand and in the wrist. Patients have a combination of ongoing moderate osteoarthritis symptoms punctuated by severe intermittent flares of chondrocalcinosis-induced pseudo-gout, which are usually managed with nonsteroidal anti-inflammatory agents and, if necessary, intra-articular corticosteroids. Hemochromatosis is diagnosed by obtaining serum iron and transferrin levels. Phlebotomy (blood letting, or removing blood) can be performed on a weekly basis and depletes the body of iron.

Patients with *hemophilia* frequently bleed into joints. The release of immense quantities of hemosiderin (iron pigment) in these patients damages cartilage and bone, and this is accompanied by eburnation of bone and osteophyte formation. This is seen to a much lesser extent in patients with *recurrent hemarthrosis* (bleeding into the joints due to other coagulation disorders) or in patients on anticoagulants, who sustain repeated trauma.

The thyroid gland, which straddles the front part of our neck, is surrounded by a series of small glands known as the parathyroid. The parathyroid gland regulates our calcium metabolism. *Hyperparathyroidism* is associated with kidney failure and a variety of metabolic conditions. Manifested by elevated serum calcium and parathormone levels, hyperparathyroid states coexist with chondrocalcinosis, osteoarthritis changes, joint aches, and pseudo-gout attacks. X-rays show subchondral bony erosions due to removal of calcium from bones. Managing the arthritis is symptomatic; many patients require removal of the gland.

In *acromegaly*, there is progressive overgrowth of soft tissue, bone, and cartilage. This is caused by hypersecretion of growth hormone by the pituitary gland. The net result is joint-space narrowing, osteophyte formation, subchondral sclerosis, and a premature osteoarthritis.

Diagnosed when patients have black urine, there is a pigment that also causes cartilage to turn black. *Ochronosis* (alkaptonuria) is a rare genetic disorder caused by deficiency of the enzyme homogentistic oxidase. It is associated with chondrocalcinosis, shards of black cartilage, spinal fusion and degeneration and early onset osteoarthritis.

Secondary osteoarthritis in patients with other forms of arthritis

Since osteoarthritis is so widespread, it is commonly seen in patients with other rheumatic disorders. Most of the time this finding is coincidental, but occasionally it can be related. Serious, ongoing, chronic inflammatory processes could be considered to be a form of trauma to the bone and can initiate premature or accelerated osteoarthritis at its areas of involvement. Examples of significant inflammation initiating an osteoarthritic response occur in bone infections, frostbite, repeated steroid injections into a joint, and rheumatoid arthritis.

Dead bones and deadened nerves producing osteoarthritis

Lauren was very athletic and sustained a severe right hip dislocation injury while on the gymnastics team of her high school. Nothing was broken, but 20 years later she began to complain of hip pain. X-rays showed accelerated osteoarthritic changes, and she was started on Relafen. Lauren also developed asthma, and her allergist had to prescribe corticosteroids. Two years later, the Relafen she took for her hip pain stopped working and the discomfort became much more severe. Repeat X-rays of her right hip demonstrated avascular necrosis (osteonecrosis). She will probably need hip surgery.

Bone requires frequent nourishment through a rich blood supply in order to grow and maintain its structural integrity. Even though cartilage is avascular (having no blood vessels), bone is not. In *avascular necrosis*, (also called osteonecrosis), cells that signal the bone to remodel osteocytes die, and new bone is not formed. The ultimate results is necrosis, or bone decay. Alternatively, oxygen supply (via blood vessels) is cut off, also causing bone death. Diagnosed on a plain X-ray in later cases or by

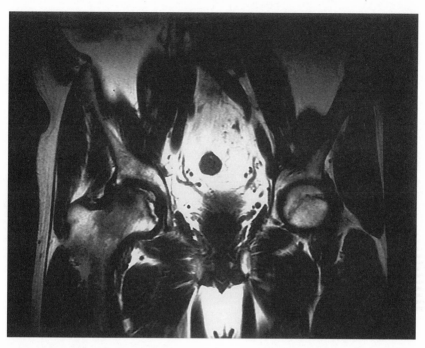

FIG. 8   *MRI showing osteonecrosis of the hip*

MRI in patients with early symptoms of pain limited to a specific area, avascular necrosis leads to osteoarthritis because the bone below the cartilage dies and the joint degenerates (illustrated in Figure 8). The most common cause of osteonecrosis is treatment with corticosteroids.

Damaged nerves decrease sensation to a particular region of the body, and may lead to altered body mechanics and localized trauma that the patient is not aware of. *Diabetes mellitus* is the most common cause of neuropathic arthropathy, followed by spinal cord injuries and advanced syphilis (an infection that affects the nervous system). Neuropathic arthropathies initially resemble osteoarthritis on X-rays with joint space narrowing, cartilage destruction, bony eburnation, tenderness, and osteophytes. Ultimately, the architecture of bone is grossly altered and one has new bone, dead bone, and bony fragments with immobilization. The primary treatment is vigilance with prophylactic foot and ankle care, appropriate bracing of the affected joint for patients with diabetic neuropathies, and control of blood sugars.

Table 7: Examples of secondary or adaptive forms of osteoarthritis

Heritable and developmental osteoarthritis
    Genetic defects producing early-onset osteoarthritis
    Endemic forms of osteoarthritis (e.g., Kashin-Beck disease)
Metabolic and hormonal forms associated with osteoarthritis
    Crystal-induced arthritis
    Hemachromatosis
    Ochronosis
    Wilson's disease (copper storage)
    Acromegaly
    Hyperparathyroidism
    Hemophilia and hemarthrosis
Osteoarthritis resulting from chronic inflammation or irritation
    Septic arthritis
    Rheumatoid arthritis
    Iatrogenic causes (frostbite, chronic steroid injections)
Important miscellaneous causes
    Neuropathic arthritis (e.g., diabetes mellitus, syphilis)
    Osteonecrosis (avascular necrosis)

SUMMARY

Ten to 15% of osteoarthritis patients develop the disease due to hormone imbalances, genetic defects, the environment, crystals, or prolonged, sustained trauma. These secondary forms of osteoarthritis also mandate attention to additional lifestyle concerns, inflammation, medication, and physical measures.

10

How Can I Be Sure It's Really Osteoarthritis?

The fact that your patient gets well does not prove that your diagnosis was correct.

—Samuel J. Meltzer (1851–1921)

Osteoarthritis is like many chronic diseases. With heart disease, for example, narrowing of the arteries begins many years before a patient develops chest pain, the chief symptom of atherosclerotic heart disease. A doctor evaluates the coronary arteries of someone with chest pain to find out how much narrowing is present. Osteoarthritis is very similar to heart disease in that articular cartilage begins to degenerate silently, and it is many years after this process has begun that a patient develops joint pain and consults a doctor. When the joint pain begins there is usually irreversible cartilage damage. However, the amount of cartilage damage at the time joint pain develops varies with each person. Some people do not develop joint pain until all of the articular cartilage has been destroyed, while others develop it very early in the disease process. However, by the time someone develops joint pain, cartilage damage has already begun.

Once joint pain from osteoarthritis begins, the course is also variable. In some people the remaining cartilage is rapidly destroyed, their joint pain becomes very severe, and they need to have a joint replacement. However, other individuals may develop pain from osteoarthritis that remains very mild for many years. All of the reasons why joints degenerate at different rates is not known, but it is the subject of intense research

61

today. This chapter will review the principal symptoms and signs of osteoarthritis, and contrast them with other rheumatic processes which
can coexist or be confused with the disorder.

THE CLINICAL PRESENTATION OF OSTEOARTHRITIS

Osteoarthritis of a joint or a number of joints has characteristic signs and
symptoms. Usually, osteoarthritis sufferers are mature adults, aged 50 or
more before symptoms start to appear. However, osteoarthritis symptoms
can appear much earlier if the patient has previously injured a joint. Patients with osteoarthritis will usually experience joint pain during or after
joint use. For example, if you have knee osteoarthritis the joint will be
painful when walking and sometimes afterwards, but not before the walk.
The symptoms are the same for the hip, back, and hands. Often, one will
experience a few minutes of joint stiffness and pain when arising in the
morning. This usually goes away in a few minutes. One may also notice
that joints swell up a little bit after using them awhile or overusing them.
These are the most common symptoms of osteoarthritis.

   If a joint is swollen, then the doctor may aspirate some joint fluid.
The joint fluid from someone with osteoarthritis usually has a few hundred inflammatory cells or some crystals, and is otherwise normal. If
blood tests are taken to try to find out if someone has another type of
arthritis, the blood tests should be normal.

Knee symptoms

Your doctor or another health care provider may perform a joint examination. If you have knee osteoarthritis, often the big muscle of the
thigh, the quadriceps muscle, may be weaker on the side of knee osteoarthritis. Also, when the doctor bends the knee you may hear some
"cracking" as your knee is put through a range of motion. This cracking
or "crepitus" results from the wearing out of the cartilage and represents
the bones at the joint rubbing against each other. Also, you may have a
little bit of joint swelling. The swelling of the knee results when the lining of the joint (the *synovium*) thickens and becomes inflamed with
more layers of cells and blood vessels. The main function of the synovium is to provide nutrition to the articular cartilage of the joint, because cartilage has no blood vessels. When the joint starts to degenerate
due to excess mechanical stresses, the synovium thickens with new blood

vessels and inflammatory cells. This may be an attempt by the joint to try to repair injured cartilage. However, thickening of the synovium leads to joint inflammation and pain. You may also notice that bones around the knee joint have grown, and fat pads that lie on both sides of the knee also thicken with osteoarthritis. The reason for fat-pad thickening is not known, but it may be another attempt by the joint to try to repair cartilage or stabilize the joint.

If the doctor obtains a X-ray of the knee, there are some characteristic findings that also help to confirm the diagnosis of osteoarthritis. First the articular cartilage between the bones of the knee joint becomes thin, so the joint space which is dark on a X-ray becomes small and the bones in the joint more closer together. This is referred to as *joint-space narrowing*. Bone spurs grow out from the margins of the bones. There can be thickening of the bone just below the joint line, and this is seen as *sclerosis* or brightness on the X-ray. Lastly, if the joint has rather advanced osteoarthritis, there may be cysts in the bone resulting from the synovium pushing into the bone, and deformities of the surrounding bones. Many stages of osteoarthritis can be seen on the radiograph. There are some very traditional ways to grade the severity of the radiograph for osteoarthritis.

It is important to know that in a disease like osteoarthritis, which can be present for many years before a patient develops any symptoms, the X-ray findings do not really correlate with the joint pain. In fact, less than 30% of individuals who have moderate findings of knee osteoarthritis by radiograph will ever have joint pain or tell their doctor about it. The reason for this lack of correspondence is not known.

Magnetic resonance imaging (MRI) has recently been used for joint imaging. A standard radiograph can only image solid structures, such as bones; soft tissues, including articular cartilage, are not seen by X-ray. An MRI takes advantage of types of magnetic field imaging and can image both hard and soft tissues. Further research will allow us to begin to answer questions about why some individuals have X-ray changes of knee osteoarthritis and joint pain, while others have X-ray changes of osteoarthritis without joint pain.

Hand osteoarthritis

Hand osteoarthritis, like knee osteoarthritis, has the same symptoms of pain during and after joint use, with a few minutes of joint stiffness in the morning. However, unlike knee osteoarthritis, individuals with hand osteoarthritis will first notice that they develop painful red bumps on their distal and middle finger joints. These painful red bumps represent the development of new bone spurs or osteophytes at the margins of the joints. The painful swelling usually goes away in a few weeks, and new bone around the finger joints is felt (Heberden's and Bouchard's nodes). The nodes characteristically develop in women about the time of menopause, and less frequently in men. On X-ray, new bone spurs are seen in the finger joint margins, there is often joint space narrowing from loss of cartilage, and some thickening of the bone underneath the joint or sclerosis. Also, the finger joint may be pushed off to one side due to joint destruction and there may be some bone cysts next to the joint.

Hip osteoarthritis

Hip osteoarthritis is very similar to knee osteoarthritis. Pain is usually experienced when walking. Occasionally pain in the hip is not noticed, but may be referred to the back or the knee. There is no way to see hip joint swelling. An X-ray of the hip will usually show joint-space narrowing, some new bone spur formation, and bone thickening or sclerosis.

HOW CAN A DOCTOR DIFFERENTIATE OSTEOARTHRITIS FROM OTHER TYPES OF ARTHRITIS?

Table 1 in chapter 1 reviewed the seven families of arthritis that account for 150 different rheumatic conditions. While many of these coexist with osteoarthritis, it is sometimes important to rule out specific diagnoses which would be treated differently than osteoarthritis.

In autoimmune conditions such as *rheumatoid arthritis, scleroderma,* and *systemic lupus erythematosus*, the body becomes allergic to itself. Although symptoms, signs, and blood testing (reviewed in chapter 8) can usually differentiate these disorders from osteoarthritis, early autoimmune disease can be mistakenly diagnosed as osteoarthritis. Patients over the age of 40 can be diagnosed with osteoarthritis (which they might also have) when it is actually rheumatoid arthritis that is evolving. Sometimes, rheumatoid arthritis presents in a subtle, slowly developing manner with morning stiffness and aching and mild joint swelling. It tends to involve the knuckles of the hands closest to the wrist which are spared in osteoarthritis. Most patients with rheumatoid arthritis have an elevated blood sedimentation rate, positive rheumatoid factor, and inflammatory joint fluid, which is not part of osteoarthritis. X-ray findings and careful clinical examination do allow for an obvious diagnosis of rheumatoid arthritis—and is important to make this diagnosis early, since the disease can be a deforming, crippling process for which prompt, aggressive intervention makes a significant impact of function and disability.

Crystal arthritis usually coexists with osteoarthritis. Over 90% of patients with pseudo-gout also have osteoarthritis, and gout is also statistically associated with osteoarthritis. Differentiated from osteoarthritis by sudden onset and the intensity of pain, these conditions are discussed in chapter 9.

Joint infections are rarely confused with osteoarthritis. Septic arthritis patients often have fevers, which are not found in osteoarthritis, and intense pain in a specific joint from which pus can be aspirated.

Metabolic bone disorders include conditions where there is too much calcium in bone (Paget's disease), not enough calcium (osteoporosis), or an abnormality in bone modeling (osteomalacia). The pain of Paget's disease can be confused with osteoarthritis, but blood testing of serum alkaline phosphatase and a close look at a patient's X-rays can usually confirm the diagnosis. Osteoporosis is not associated with pain unless a fracture is also present, which usually can be readily seen on a X-ray.

Soft tissue rheumatism involves the supporting structure of joints, such as the tendons, bursae, or ligaments. They are frequently associated with osteoarthritis and its management can be similar. Localized manifestations of fibromyalgia can be aggravated by osteoarthritis in the area, but this syndrome does not affect joints.

Seronegative spondyloarthropathies such as ankylosing spondylitis, reactive arthritis, psoriatic arthritis, and the arthritis of inflammatory bowel disease frequently comingle with osteoarthritis. Many of these patients have rashes, a positive blood test for the HLA-B27 marker, as well as specific X-ray findings unique to this family of diseases. These include sacroilitis, ensethitis, and bony erosions.

SUMMARY

Osteoarthritis is a slowly evolving process that is usually biochemically evident years before it is diagnosed. The clinical symptoms and signs vary slightly depending upon the joint involved. Osteoarthritis can co-exist with other arthritic diseases, and its management may involve treating more than one condition. Certain forms of arthritis, such as rheumatoid arthritis, need to be ruled out to prevent crippling, deforming disease.

Part IV

HOW AND WHERE CAN THE BODY BE AFFECTED BY OSTEOARTHRITIS?

The chronical (arthritis) differs from acute rheumatism . . . with little or no fever, in having a duller pain . . . but the swellings are more permanent, and the disease of much longer duration . . . Both kinds of rheumatism attack indiscriminately males and females, rich and poor.

—William Heberden,
Commentaries on the History and Cure of Diseases (1802)

When osteoarthritis attacks the knees, is it different than when it occurs in the back? The answer is yes. We don't have discs in our knees or menisci in our back. As a result, osteoarthritis has many different "moods" as it appears in different parts of the body. Many of us walk miles a day on our feet or lift things with our shoulders—and the authors of this book spend a great deal of time typing on computer keyboards. Chapters 11 and 12 detail how arthritis affects and influences the function of different parts of the body, while chapter 13 discusses how unique mechanical considerations in specific regions of the body (among other factors) lead to certain distinct subsets or off-shoots of osteoarthritis.

11

The Upper Body and Extremities

Whoever named it necking was a poor judge of anatomy.
—Groucho Marx (1890–1977)

The body has one hundred joints, and some of them are found in unlikely places, such as the cricoarytenoid joint in the larynx. Not all of these joints are susceptible to osteoarthritic changes, and some are involved infrequently. This chapter will focus on the temporomandibular (TMJ or jaw), sternal, shoulder, elbow, wrist, and hand joints.

ARTHRITIC JAWS

Because of jaw pain, John had a great deal of difficulty chewing meat and finally consulted his dentist. He had injured the area several years before and also had a tendency to grind his teeth. X-rays revealed evidence for right temporomandibular joint osteoarthritis. He was given ibuprofen, a bite guard, and a muscle relaxant to use at bedtime. Within a month, the discomfort had greatly decreased, and he only occasionally needed medicine.

The jaw is a lay term describing the temporomandibular joints, or TMJ. The TMJ represents the articulation of the temporal tubercle with the condyle of the mandible. The synovial lining of the joint may become inflamed in rheumatoid arthritis. This is especially the case

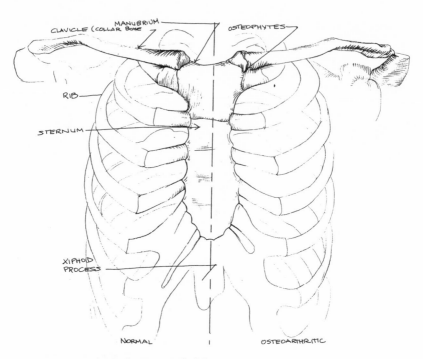

FIG. 9   *Sterno-clavicular osteoarthritis*

among adolescents with juvenile rheumatoid arthritis. Ten million Americans complain of jaw discomfort and are diagnosed with "temporomandibular joint dysfunction syndrome." The overwhelming majority of these individuals simply have muscular spasm in the area, and many also have fibromyalgia. A small number develop osteoarthritic changes in the joint. Patients may complain of muscle spasms while chewing, and cracking sounds when opening and closing their mouth. The jaws usually look normal, but on examination, the bite may be off kilter. Usually, doctors do not worry if they can place two of their fingers in the patient's mouth without producing pain. TMJ osteoarthritis is managed with nonsteroidal anti-inflammatory agents, exercises, local injections, and specialized bite guards. Surgery is rarely necessary.

STERNAL (BREAST BONE) JOINTS

The breastbone, or sternum, has articulations with the manubrium and clavicle, or collarbone (Figure 9) and is connected to the ribs. These

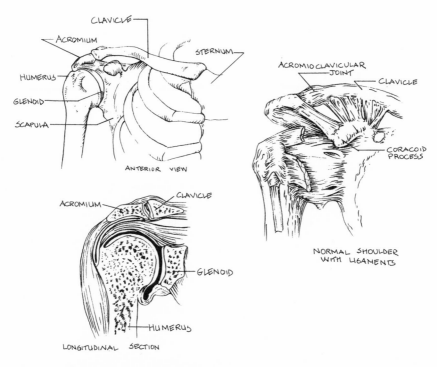

FIG. 10   *Three views of the shoulder joint*

joints are rarely affected by osteoarthritis. Most patients with osteoarthritic findings in this area have had previous trauma to or infections in the joint area.

SHOULDERING ITS BURDEN

Consisting of the clavicle (collarbone), scapula (shoulder blade), and
humerus, the shoulder is a ball-and-socket joint. The head of the
humerus is a perfect sphere, allowing a shallow, gliding broad range of
motion. It connects to the glenoid of the scapula, which acts as an anchor for upper limb muscles. The clavicle, in turn, is a long and slender
bone with connections to the acromium and sternum (Figure 10). The
shoulder region is a complex construct of muscles, ligaments, and tendons. The supraspinatus, infraspinatus, and teres minor muscles form
the *rotator cuff*, which lifts and internally and externally rotates the
humerus. Medium to large muscles from the back (trapezius, serratius

anterior, pectoralis major, and biceps) stabilize the shoulder blade and allow upper arm motions. Upper arm strength and leverage is provided by
the deltoid, pectoralis minor, teres major, and lattisimus dorsi muscles.
The shoulder region joints (glenohumeral, acromioclavicular, sterno-
clavicular, and scapulothoracic) work together to promote upper extremity motion.

Osteoarthritis is uncommon in the shoulder. When diagnosed, it is
usually a consequence of trauma, overuse, or chronic inflammation.

> When Troy attended college, he pitched for the baseball team. Although he
> was not good enough to hope to make the major leagues, he played semi-
> pro ball while building up his plumbing supply business. By the time he
> was 40, his shoulder hurt so much he could barely lift pipes. His doctor
> found evidence for acromioclavicular joint arthritis and a glemohumeral
> bursitis. Dr. Metzger told him that pitching had damaged his joint, in-
> jected his bursa with a cortisone/xylocaine combination, prescribed cele-
> coxib (Celebrex), and initiated a shoulder rehabilitation program.

The shoulder examination

When a health care professional first evaluates a shoulder complaint,
they first look at the joint. Is it swollen, red, or atrophied? The shoulder
region is then examined by touch. Is warmth, tenderness, or inflammation present? Could the pain be from the joint, bursa, tendon, or a ligament? Frequently, pain radiates to the shoulder from the neck. Ulnar
and median nerves in the lower cervical and upper thoracic spine can
transmit neck pain to the shoulder region. Subscapular or long thoracic
nerve and brachial plexus neuropathies emanate from the neck but produce discomfort in the shoulder region. In other words, osteoarthritis of
the cervical spine is one of the most common causes of shoulder pain.
Could associated muscular spasm be associated with fibromyalgia or regional myofascial pain syndrome? The biceps tendon should be palpated, since inflammation of it is common. *Ligamentitis* (an inflamed
ligament) is common in the shoulder and areas supporting the
acromioclavicular, coracoacromion, coracoclavicular, sternoclavicular,
glenohumeral, and coracohumeral ligaments should be felt. Finally, the
shoulder is moved in a variety of directions: forward flexion (to 90 degrees), backward extension (to 45 degrees), abduction (to 180 degrees),
adduction (to 45 degrees), external rotation (to 40-45 degrees) and in-

ternal rotation (to 55 degrees). Motions of the glenohumeral joint and rotator cuff are given special attention. How well does the shoulder move when observed from both the front and back? Can the joint move actively, or does it assume certain positions only when passively guided there (as in a partial rotator cuff tear)? Is the joint stable?

Conditions associated with osteoarthritis of the shoulder

> George worked in construction. He was very skilled at manipulating a pulley which required him to lift 40 pounds at a time while operating levers necessitating repeated shoulder rotation. After doing this for 15 years, George's shoulder started to hurt. X-rays showed joint-space narrowing consistent with osteoarthritis and his physical examination additionally suggested a partial rotator cuff tear. The latter was injected with corticosteroids and Dr. Shadwick prescribed Vioxx for the osteoarthritis. An occupational and physical therapy program taught George strengthening exercises and how to limit further damage. His boss gave him a supervisory job and hopefully, surgery can be avoided.

Figure 11 demonstrates where osteoarthritis of the shoulder may occur. Its symptoms are often poorly localized. For example, acromioclavicular osteoarthritis is rarely associated with tenderness in that area, and its pain is referred elsewhere. The bursa, tendons, and ligaments around the rotator cuff surround the glenohumeral joint. Arthritis changes in the joint are associated with altered range of motion, mediated by the cuff. Failure to adequately move the shoulder due to pain may cause the joint to "freeze" or become immobile. This "joint freezing" is known as *adhesive capsulitis*, this usually correlates with impingement of the subacromial bursa and supraspinatus muscle between the top of the humerus. Rotator cuff tears can be partial or complete, and usually produce tendinitis. Calcium deposits (which can crystallize and result in a situation much like pseudo-gout) are common in inflamed tendons. Bone spurs in the shoulder joint lead to altered biomechanics and subsequent *subacromial* and *subscapular bursitis*. Shoulder osteoarthritis is managed with vigorous exercise and rehabilitation programs, acetaminophen, nonsteroidal anti-inflammatory drugs, and local injections. Arthroscopy is a surgical procedure where an operating telescope/microscope is placed into the shoulder and an orthopedist can repair tears,

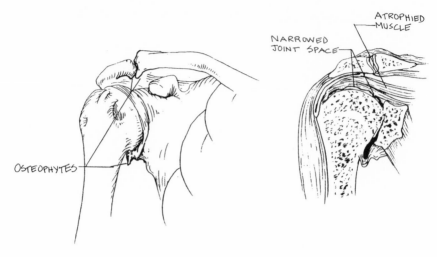

FIG. 11   *Osteoarthritis of the shoulder*

dissolve calcium deposits, and help free up adhesions. Open-shoulder surgery for osteoarthritis is rarely recommended.

THE ELBOW

The elbow is a hinge joint consisting of three bones: the humerus, radius, and ulna (Figure 12). It has three articulations: humeral-ulnar, radio-humeral, and proximal radio-ulnar, which permit arm flexion and normal use. Normal extension is only 0-5 degrees, while flexion up to 135 degrees is allowed. The elbow is surrounded by several bursae; the olecrenon in particular can fill up with fluid when pressure is placed on the area. Most elbow pathology is related to its epicondyles or bony configurations where muscles, ligaments, and tendons attach. Inflammation of the medial epicondyle (golf elbow) or lateral epicondyle (tennis elbow, from carrying briefcases or portfolios) is not usually associated with osteoarthritis. Osteoarthritis of the elbow joint is seen in weight lifters and pitchers, and after an injury, but is uncommon. When present, it can result in flexion deformities. Swelling in the elbow joint suggests rheumatoid arthritis. Rheumatoid nodules may be palpable through the skin. Elbow osteoarthritis is managed locally with anti-inflammatory medication, exercises, or local injections. Surgery is rarely advised.

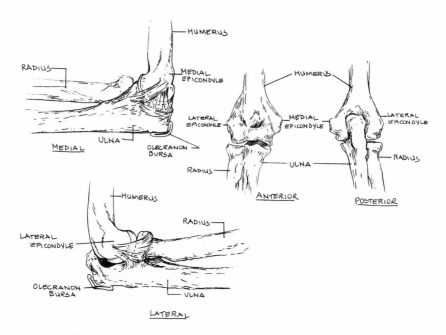

FIG. 12A   *The elbow joint*

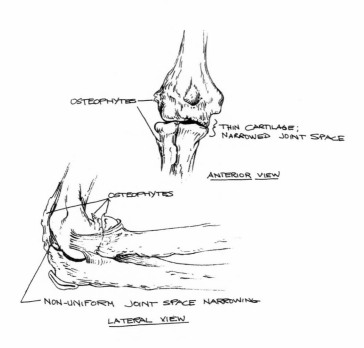

FIG. 12B   *Osteoarthritis of the elbow*

THE WRIST AND HAND

Jeri noticed pain at the outer area of her right wrist, which spread to the base of her right thumb. At rest it did not bother her, but whenever she knitted or wrote for more than a few minutes, it throbbed. In the morning, it felt stiff and achy before she showered. X-rays of the hand and wrist demonstrated osteoarthritis of the carpometacarpal, or CMC joint. Dr. Janes explained to her that this was a common area of osteoarthritis involvement. Advil upset her stomach, so Dr. Janes prescribed Celebrex as needed, and a CMC splint to use with knitting or writing.

The wrist and hand complex consist of 27 bones. Acting as the chief "sensory organ" of the body, it permits grasping, dressing, eating, reaching, writing, and personal hygiene. The wrist contains eight carpal bones in two rows, which act as ball bearings, facilitate rotary movements, and articulate with the radius (Figure 13). This gives way to five rays (our fingers) connected by hinge, or tongue-and-groove joints. Covered by extrinsic muscles from the forearm and intrinsic muscles within the hand, our fingers are able to flex (bend), extend (straighten), and abduct (move apart). The metacarpophalangeal (MCP), proximal interphalangeal (PIP), and distal interphalangeal (DIP) joints are held in place by tendons and ligaments. The most complicated articulation is the thumb. This saddle-shaped joint is a focal area involved in osteoarthritis, and its rotary movements are supported by eight separate muscles and tendons.

The wrist and hand examination

Inspecting the wrist and hand can identify cysts, deformities, thick tendons, calcium deposits, swelling (as in rheumatoid arthritis), Raynaud's syndrome (where fingers turn different colors in cold weather), nail pitting (seen in psoriatic arthritis), clubbing (downward motion of the nails observed in certain lung diseases), and muscle wasting. Nodules or nodes can also be seen. Rheumatoid arthritis commonly involves the near and middle knuckles (MCPs and PIPs), whereas osteoarthritis involves the middle and far knuckles (PIPs and DIPs). Palpation of the joints can confirm the character of cysts, calcium deposits, gouty tophi, inflammation of the synovium, or tightness of the skin (as in sclero-

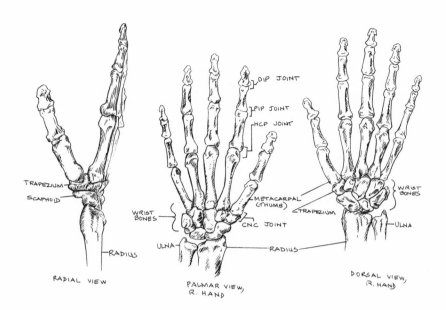

FIG. 13A   *The hand wrist*

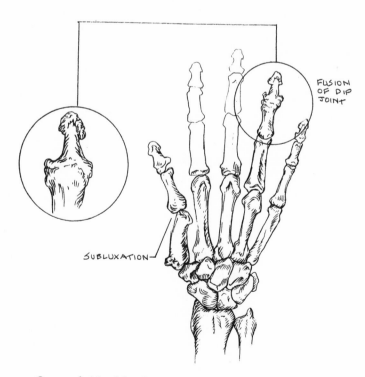

FIG. 13B   *Osteoarthritis of the CMC and hand joints*

derma). Movements of the fingers and wrist (60-70 degrees of extension and 80-90 degrees of flexion) may demonstrate contractures, inflammation of tendons, and numbness or tingling sensations (as in carpal tunnel syndrome). Grip strength and fine motor movement functions are ultimately evaluated.

Osteoarthritis of the hand and wrist

Eight percent of adults in the United States have moderate to severe osteoarthritis of the hands. Most of these individuals have carpometacarpal (CMC) arthritis, or changes at the trapezium (a carpal bone)-metacarpal joint (see Figure 13). Located in the thumb region, patients complain of painful motions, and have decreased joint stability. CMC arthritis is treated with splinting, acetaminophen, anti-inflammatory regimens, and local injections. Surgery is infrequently called for. Osteoarthritic changes in the other carpal bones is uncommon. In our senior citizens, osteoarthritic changes are found in the following joints: DIP 70%, PIP 35%, MCP 15%, CMC 50%, and wrist 12%.

The other common area of osteoarthritis involvement is at the PIP and DIP joints. Often painless, these hereditary nodules usually form in the fourth decade of life, and affect females in a 10:1 ratio. Known as Bouchard's (PIP) and Hebreden's (DIP) nodes, they may be associated with hand pain for the first year of two after they form, and usually appear as asymptomatic deformities thereafter. Nonsteroidal or acetominophen medication is the treatment of choice. Corticosteroid injections may be helpful in early cases, and surgery is usually not indicated.

Osteoarthritis of the wrist and hands may occur with a variety of conditions. These include *carpal tunnel syndrome*, where nerves traversing through the wrist to the hands are compressed, producing numbness and tingling in the first, second, third, and the "thumb" side of the fourth finger. Repetitive motions such as typing or lifting can cause this. Thick contractures of the palmar fascia, producing flexion deformities of the fourth and fifth fingers, are seen in diabetics and in other conditions. Termed a *Dupuytren's contracture*, this painful condition is often difficult to treat. Inflammation of the tendon sheaths at the base of the thumb near the radial styloid is called *de Quervain's tenosynovitis*, which can be hard to differentiate from CMC osteoarthritis and coexists with it. Sometimes osteoarthritis of an area may alter the biomechanics of a tendon, producing a locking or "trigger finger" effect. Early on, local injections usually successfully manage de Quervain's tenosynoritis. Infrequently, severe osteoarthritis changes of the finger are associated with nerve entrapments, ligamentitis, tendonitis, or local ruptures.

SUMMARY

Osteoarthritis of the elbow and shoulder are uncommon and are usually associated with trauma or overuse. Osteoarthritis commonly affects the DIP and PIP joints in the wrist and hand, but is more disfiguring than painful in these locations. Carpometacarpal arthritis can be quite uncomfortable and function limiting.

12

The Spine

Its Nooks and Tingles

Grief never mended no broken bones.
> —Charles Dickens (1812–1870),
> *Sketches by Boz*

Appreciating how elegantly humans are functionally structured creates a feeling of awe. Perhaps such a design could only have been crafted by a higher source. The longest bony structure of the body, the spine, provides stability, mobility, outlets for nearly all of our nerves, protection, rigidity, and distinguishes us from other mammals with its erectness. It allows us to move, function, and feel sensations. In this chapter, you will learn how the spine is constructed, the means by which doctors examine it, which diagnostic studies evaluate symptoms, and how different types of osteoarthritis affect it.

BONING UP: A FUNCTIONAL ANATOMY LESSON

Our spine consists of 33 separate *vertebrae*. They are divided into five regions based on their appearance: cervical, or neck (7 bones); thoracic (12); lumbar (5), sacral (5 vertebrae, usually fused together); and coccyx (4 fused segments). The vertebrae increase in size consecutively from the second cervical through the sacral region, after which they become smaller. Interconnected by muscles, discs, cartilage, and ligaments, the spine has four curvatures: (the cervical and lumbar, which look concave and produce lordosis; and the thoracic and sacral, which look convex and produce kyphosis). These support weight-bearing and act as a single column. These contractures allow flexibility, rotation, bending, compression, movement, and loading.

Discs separate the vertebrae, and contain fibrous tissue and cartilage that act as shock absorbers. Connecting peripheral signals to the central nervous system of the brain, and relaying signals from the brain to the rest of the body via a doughnut-like hole in the center of the vertebrae, is the *spinal cord* (Figure 14). The spinal cord is encased in a sac or "wrapping" known as the *dura*, around which is spinal fluid. Nerves and blood vessels emanate from the spinal cord through holes in the side of the vertebrae known as *foramen* (Figure 15). This comprises the peripheral nervous system. From C1 to S4 via a *dermatomal* distribution, they are the nerve supply to the arms, legs, trunk, and reproductive areas (Figure 16).

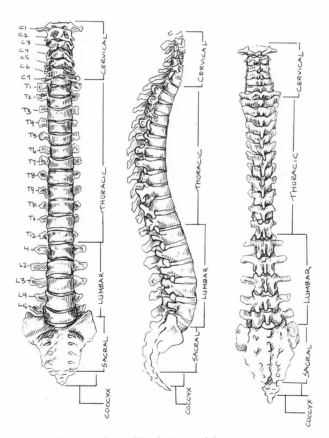

FIG. 14   *Front, side, and back views of the spine*

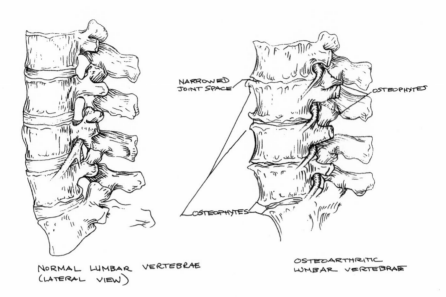

NORMAL LUMBAR VERTEBRAE
(LATERAL VIEW)

NARROWED
JOINT SPACE

OSTEOPHYTES

OSTEOPHYTES

OSTEOARTHRITIC
LUMBAR VERTEBRAE

FIG. 15A   *Normal lumbar vertebrae and osteoarthritic lumbar vertebrae*

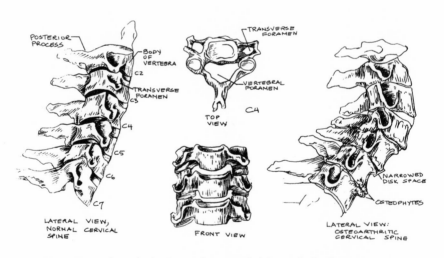

POSTERIOR
PROCESS

BODY
OF
VERTEBRA

C2

TRANSVERSE
FORAMEN
C3

C4

C5

C6

C7

LATERAL VIEW,
NORMAL CERVICAL
SPINE

TRANSVERSE
FORAMEN

VERTEBRAL
FORAMEN

C4

TOP
VIEW

FRONT VIEW

NARROWED
DISK SPACE

OSTEOPHYTES

LATERAL VIEW:
OSTEOARTHRITIC
CERVICAL SPINE

FIG. 15B   *Normal cervical spine and osteoarthritic cervical spine*

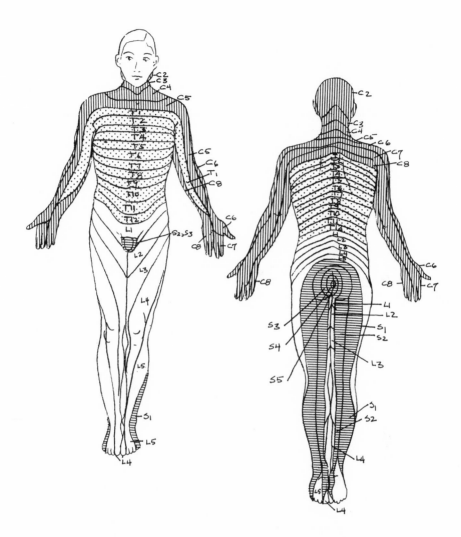

FIG. 16A   *Dermatomes: skin regions innervated by spinal nerves*

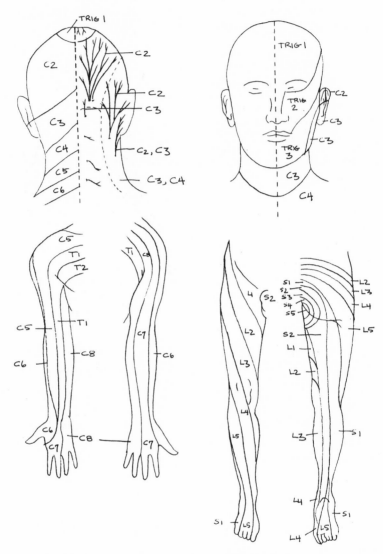

FIG. 16B   *Dermatomes: skin regions innervated by spinal nerves*

The rear or posterior portion of vertebrae looks like a series of tails or scales, and are termed *spinous processes*. Similar pouchings are found on both sides, which are termed *transverse processes*. Two "hooks" or *facets* (apophyseal joints) on the top and bottom of most vertebrae act as the glue which attaches them to each other and gives a "stacked" appearance.

Functionally, the spine protects the spinal cord. At the top is the cervical spine, which supports and allows motion of the head. In this area are several unique features. Here, the transverse processes have holes through which blood vessels traverse. Also, in the upper cervical spine are *joints of Luschka* which are lined by synovium. This tissue covering can easily become inflamed in disorders such as rheumatoid arthritis and ankylosing spondylitis. Last, the first and second cervical vertebrae (known as the atlas and axis) have a unique structure. The atlas lacks a vertebral body, but the configuration permits nodding and lateral bending of the neck. The thoracic spine is splinted by costovertebral joints, which extend to the ribs and limit motion. Pain from this region is uncommon. The lumbar spine takes weight from the upper part of the body but has less facility for movement. The sacrum and coccyx are essentially motionless, but are subject to minor manipulations by local ligaments and muscles.

I HAVE PAIN IN THE BACK. WHAT SHOULD MY DOCTOR DO?

If you seek consultation from a musculoskeletal specialist for back pain, your visit should start with a medical history. How long have you had the pain? Where exactly is it? Who has been consulted (e.g., a neurologist, an orthopedic specialist, or a rheumatologist)? What activities or motions make it better or worse? What non-medicinal treatments have been tried? (These might include physical therapy, chiropractic therapy, exercise, psychotherapy, biofeedback, acupuncture, or over-the-counter remedies such as homeopathic preparations, herbs, and vitamins.) What prescription medicines have been used? In what dose and for what length were they given and did they help? What side effects occurred?

At this point, a physical examination should be performed. The practitioner first inspects the spine for postural abnormalities such as scoliosis or stooping, blemishes, or evidence of malnutrition. Next, the spine is usually touched from top to bottom to look for painful areas. Fractures, tumors, and herniated discs, for example, can elicit signs of discomfort. The adjacent muscles and fascia around the spine are also palpated. Localized areas of tenderness can indicate injury, fibromyalgia, strain, or inflammation. The motions of the neck and lumbar spine are assessed by asking you to flex, extend, or rotate certain areas. Motion against resistance allows your doctor to see how strong your muscles are. Pulses and reflexes in your arms and legs are checked, and if abnormal, may point to vascular or nerve problems. Sometimes specific maneuvers help your doctor make a diagnosis. For example, a positive "straight leg raising" test (indicating pain in the back of the leg while raising it,) might suggest the presence of a herniated lumbar disc, while the inability to bend forward and touch your toes, with pain on palpating the sacroiliac joint, could indicate ankylosing spondylitis. Patients might be asked to walk on their heels or toes to assess muscle strength or look for atrophy.

THE SPECTRUM OF BACK PAIN

Back pain is a major public health problem. Ten to 20% of the population in the United States complains of some form of back or neck pain each year. Sixty-five to 80% of us will have low back pain or neck pain in our lifetime. Back discomfort is the fifth most common reason for seeing a physician, accounting for over two million office visits a year. Spinal pain is the most common cause of disability in patients under the age of 45. Though 5-10 billion dollars a year are spent on diagnosing and treating spinal disorders, its cumulative cost to society, including disability and litigation, is somewhere between 25 and 100 billion dollars annually. When the causes of back pain are factored into these figures, mechanical back pain is found in 90% of patients, with systemic diseases accounting for the remaining 10%.

SYMPTOMS OF NECK AND LOW BACK PAIN

In chapter 7, we reviewed the primary complaints that an osteoarthritis patient reports to their doctor. When these are narrowed down to those who have neck, mid-, or low back pain, what is usually bothering them? The most common symptom is pain, especially localized discomfort, which may be focal, encompass a specific region of the body, or radiate in a nerve-like distribution down an arm or leg. If this is associated with fever, fatigue, or weight loss, systemic conditions or disorders with abnormal blood tests should be sought out. We often ask the patient about the character of the pain. Is it continuous or intermittent? Is it deep or superficial? Does it hurt when touched? Is it boring, searing,

associated with numbness or tingling? Based on the patient's complaints, our questions, the physical examination, laboratory testing, X-
rays, and other imaging studies or electrical studies, pain in the low
back and neck can be diagnosed and classified as shown in Table 8
(at the end of the chapter). Those associated with osteoarthritis will be
discussed in detail.

GENERALIZED OSTEOARTHRITIS IN THE BACK AND NECK

Sylvia's left upper back started hurting. Whenever she lifted something heavier than 10 pounds or jumped as part of her exercise program, a shooting sensation went from her neck towards the shoulder
along the back. Dr. Campos thought it might be related to a localized
fibromyalgia or shoulder problem, but when she obtained X-rays, it
was impinging into Sylvia's neuroforamen, where her C5 spinal nerve
was found. A large osteophytic bone spur was causing the problem.
Sylvia was given a cervical collar to wear for a few weeks, started on
Naprosyn, and taught cervical isometrics (strengthening exercises
that do not involve moving the neck). The pain eased up, and Sylvia
only occasionally needs medication.

The symptoms of osteoarthritis (reviewed in chapter 7) are also found
in the neck and back areas. These include stiffness, aching, and pain.
The transverse processes, facets, and spinous processes can get bigger,
develop osteophytes, and make foramens or openings smaller. Joint-
space narrowing between the vertebrae is common as our discs degenerate with time. The intervetebral disc is composed of a tough outer shell
known as the *annulus fibrosis* and a soft semiliquid center, which binds
large amounts of water called the *nucleus pulposus*. With aging and traumatic stresses, the outer layer cracks and its integrity becomes compromised. The disc space narrows, and the semiliquid center can leak or
herniate out from its capsule. As a consequence, localized inflammation
and irritation can cause discomfort. This stimulates the formation of
osteophytes. These bone spurs can touch nerves, which produce a burning, shooting, or tingling sensation. Sometimes they impact upon ligaments or muscles in the area. With time the structural anatomy of the

region is altered, which affects posture, body mechanics, and strength. (Examples of this are shown in Figure 15.)

In the neck, most degenerative changes are found in the lower cervical spine. When the upper neck is involved, neck pain and headaches from the back of the head are common. Sometimes patients complain of dizziness. Since nerves from the fourth to seventh cervical vertebra go to the shoulders and arms, bone spurs, which press upon nerves, can produce pain in these areas (Table 9, at the end of the chapter). The amount of pain and function depends on the degree of compression. Compressive neuropathies can be occasional, positional, continuous, mild, moderate, or severe. Usually one-sided (a bone spur in the exact center would go to both sides), untreated nerve impingement can lead to muscle atrophy, weakness, and chronic shooting pain to various regions of the upper extremities. Most of us show osteoarthritic changes on plain X-rays in our neck as we age. However, not everybody who has abnormal X-rays or obvious arthritic changes on examination has symptoms. In fact, though X-ray changes are evident in back or neck films in 60% of all Americans over the age of 60, a minority of them have any symptoms or complaints. Among those with symptoms, diagnostic studies can be ordered to ascertain if the radiographic changes are of any clinical significance. These include the MRI scans, CT scans, and electrical studies (EMG and nerve conduction studies) discussed in chapter 8.

Osteoarthritis of the thoracic spine is occasionally identified on X-ray, but is an uncommon cause of any symptoms. *Scoliosis* is a curvature of the spine in excess of 10 degrees. It most commonly begins in adolescence, and produces back and regional myofascial pain due to poor posture. These changes lead to accelerated or early osteoarthritis in the middle and low back.

Those who have symptoms of arthritis emanating from the lumbar spine, or low back, fall into one of three categories. There may be instability of the spinal column, malalignment of the spinal column, or a tightening of the nerve roots as they leave the spinal canal. This in turn is associated with different types of pain. For example, instability of the column might result in a dull, boring back discomfort. Tightening of the nerve roots (as in sciatica) causes a sharp, radiating, electrical-like pain. If pain in the legs is crampy, intermittent, and associated with activity, most doctors would be concerned about blood flow and circulation. However, if the crampy pain is limited to the upper legs and is relieved with bending forward, spinal stenosis should be considered.

Spondylosis and spondylolisthesis

Al had a vague ache in his low back. It seemed a bit worse on the left side, and sometimes travelled to his buttock but never went down the leg. The pain worsened with bending over. Dr. Prager found no real abnormalities on Al's physical examination. Range of motion, pulses, reflexes, and strength was normal. An X-ray demonstrated some slippage in the lumbar region with mild to moderate osteoarthritic changes. The L4 vertebral body moved forward compared to the next lower one. Al was told to lose weight, given an abdominal muscle strengthening exercise program, and instructed to take up to eight Tylenol a day when the pain became uncomfortable. When he gardens, he uses a lumbar band for support.

This form of back and neck pain usually produces localized discomfort or none at all. Diagnosed by X-rays of the spine, which show degenerative changes, *spondylosis* is the consequence of intersegmental instability due to a stress fracture of two small bones, resulting from shifts in compressive forces between facets and intervertebral discs (Figure 17). Pain

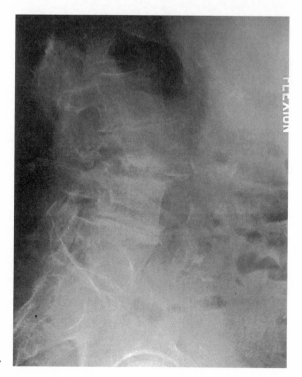

FIG. 17A *Lumbar spondylosis, lateral view*

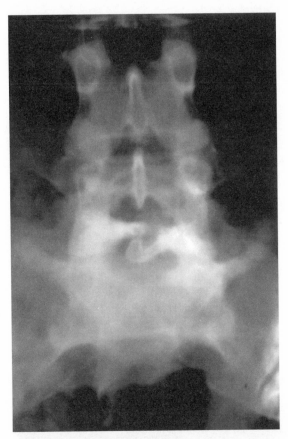

FIG. 17B *Posterior view*

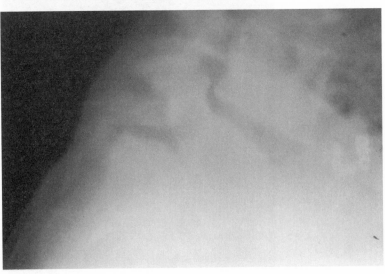

FIG. 17C *L4-5 spondylolisthesis*

may worsen with extension, but no neurologic deficits are present. Acetaminophen helps mild pain, and nonsteroidal anti-inflammatory agents relieve mild to moderate symptoms.

As spondylosis evolves, the vertebral body may become displaced or lean forward, resulting in a crooked spine, or *spondylolisthesis*. Degenerative spondylolisthesis is usually seen at the L4-L5 lumbar level and is associated with degenerative disc disease and disease of the facet joints, leading to segmental instability. A stress fracture of the pars intra-articularis is responsible for this. Low back pain is worse with standing and relieved by rest. Neurologic symptoms are absent, though fusion surgery may be required if the slippage becomes neurologically compromising.

What is a herniated disc?

> Elyse woke up three weeks ago with a piercing pain in her right buttock area that went down the back of her thigh and the front of her shin. When she tried to get up, she found herself unable to stand without feeling an unbearable stabbing sensation in her right leg. Her husband drove her to Urgent Care, where a diagnosis of acute sciatica was made. Elyse was placed at bedrest for three days with a hot pack under her back and pillows under her knees. She took Tylenol with codeine every six hours so that she could sit up and eat and go to the bathroom. Her condition eventually eased up. Though X-rays of her lumbar spine demonstrated a few osteoarthritic changes, an MRI showed a large herniated disc. Elyse is undergoing a rehabilitation program and is taking Vioxx along with a muscle relaxant at bed time. Though it has been three weeks, she is now 80% improved and has returned to work.

When disc material extrudes from the nucleus pulposus and touches adjacent nerves, we are said to have a herniated disc. In the neck this can lead to numbness, and there may also be tingling in the shoulders, forearms, and hands known as *radicular symptoms* (see Table 9). Neck pain can be minimal or absent, and complaints are brought on by heavy exertion or lifting. We usually initially give these patients nonsteroidals, local injections, or a cervical collar if indicated, and reduce their activities. Unlike the cervical or lumbar discs, clinically urgent herniated thoracic discs are almost unheard of, and intervention is required in very few instances. Such is not the case for the lower back regions; herniated lumbar discs are common, and produce radicular symptoms in the lower extremity.

Most disc herniations occur in the L4-L5 and L5-S1 vertebral region, producing *sciatica,* or irritation of the sciatic nerve. The largest nerve in the body, sciatica is associated with a painful numbing and shooting sensation down the back of the buttock, thigh, and in more advanced cases the front of the lower leg, and side of the foot. Identified by a positive straight leg raising test, sciatica is managed acutely with bed rest, anti-inflammatory drugs, and local injections of corticosteroids or epidural blocks if necessary, where corticosteroids are placed in the epidural space. While lying down, the patients knees should be supported by pillows, and sitting, bending over, or stooping should be restricted. Untreated or incompletely treated herniated discs result in muscle atrophy, loss of reflexes, and weakness.

Though infrequent, sacral nerve compression can occur. Since the sacral nerves innervate our reproductive tract, bladder, and anus, involvement of this region can produce a *cauda equina syndrome,* characterized by inability to urinate or defecate. This is an orthopedic or neurosurgical emergency.

Since spinal stenosis, fibromyalgia, whiplash, neck or low back strain, and a variety of other conditions may be confused with a herniated disc, the diagnosis can be definitively made with a MRI or CT scan of the affected region (Figure 18). Evidence for "bulging of the disc" on an imaging report (which is common) rarely produces symptoms. If there is any question as to the nature and degree of how the abnormality is affecting function of a nerve or muscle, an EMG or nerve conduction can assess this quantitatively.

WHAT IS SPINAL STENOSIS?

Leon began noticing a toothache-like painful sensation in his thighs. It was dull, persistent, and annoying. Neither Tylenol, aspirin, nor Advil helped. He saw his family doctor. Dr. Steen's physical examination was normal, and X-rays of the lumbar spine showed only mild degenerative changes. Dr. Steen ordered a blood panel with arthritis tests as well as an EMG and nerve conduction to look for evidence of a muscle or nerve root problem. All were normal. Leon's discomfort

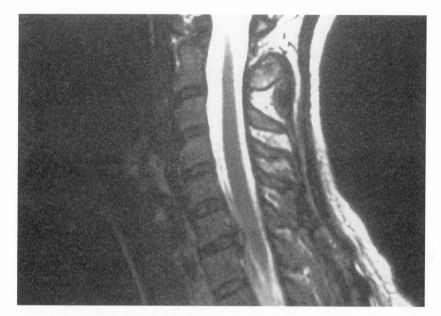

FIG. 18A   *MRI of lumbar spine showing a herniated disc, lateral view*

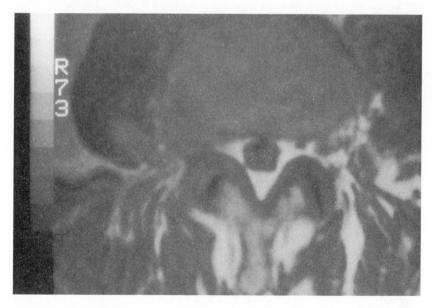

FIG. 18B   *Frontal view*

increased. Physical therapy was of little benefit. A corticosteroid shot into the left hip made no difference. Neither codeine nor Darvon were able to control the pain. Leon seemed to feel better when he bent over. Finally, an MRI was performed which revealed a tight spinal stenosis. After 3 weekly epidural corticosteroid injections, Leon experienced relief for the first time. Hopefully, surgery won't be necessary.

Spinal stenosis could not be diagnosed pre-operatively before 1975, when CT scanning became readily available. Defined as a narrowing of the openings through which nerves exit the spinal canal, this tightening or narrowing stenosis can be present at birth (congenital spinal stenosis) and evident in our early years. Spinal stenosis associated with osteoarthritis results from the growth of osteophytes and posterior bulging of the intervetebral discs, causing pressure on the spinal cord (Figure 19). The symptoms of spinal stenosis develop insidiously. Cervical stenosis is often congenital; thoracic stenosis almost never is a problem. Lumbar spinal stenosis produces a dull aching in the upper legs that the patient rarely associates with a back problem, and they often challenge the physician who proposes taking lumbar spine X-rays. Leg

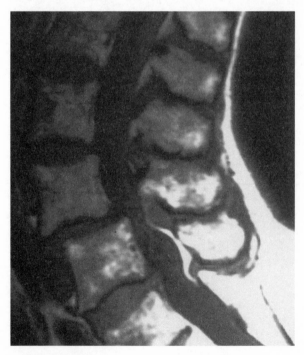

FIG. 19   *MRI of lumbar spine showing spinal stenosis*

pain appears with activity but can be relieved by sitting or flexing forward, which increases room in the spinal canal and improves blood flow. X-rays may show disc degeneration, but cannot by themselves make a diagnosis of spinal stenosis. CT scans or MRI scans are usually necessary to make the diagnosis of spinal canal narrowing. Spinal stenosis due to osteoarthritis tends to become symptomatic in one's 70s and 80s, when aggressive management is often neither desired nor often possible. Nonsteroidals are mildly helpful, and epidural corticosteroid injections can provide months to years of relief in most cases. Decompressive neurosurgery is usually curative and surprisingly well-tolerated. Necessitating only two to three days of hospitalization, it has a very high success rate and few complications. Untreated spinal stenosis rarely compresses the spinal cord to the point where weakness, incoordination, spasticity, and peculiar sensations result. Known as a *myelopathy,* this serious condition can produce lasting nerve damage or even quadriplegia or paraplegia (paralysis) if it is not aggressively managed.

YES, THERE IS A VARIANT OF OSTEOARTHRITIS WITH A SILLY NAME: DISH

In the early 1900s, Jacques Forestier described a form of osteoarthritis characterized by large bone spurs, marginal bone formation, and calcification of ligaments. Occurring mostly in the spine, *diffuse idiopathic skeletal hyperostosis* (DISH, also known as ankylosing hyperostosis or Forestier's disease) tends to occur in middle aged men. Diagnosed in X-rays (Figure 20), it usually causes no symptoms and can be seen in patients taking retinoid (Vitamin A derivative) medicines and in diabetics. Occasionally DISH can produce stiffness, difficulty swallowing (when the osteophytes press on the back of the esophagus), and decreased spinal mobility. Nonsteroidals are usually helpful.

SUMMARY

Thirty-three bones in our spine function as a locomotion unit, providing balance, erectness, strength, and support for nerve function. With age and wear and tear, the neck and low back regions, in particular, evolve degenerative changes which can produce pain, weakness, and

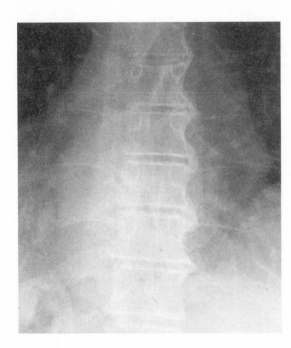

FIG. 20   *Calicification of spinal ligaments producing DISH*

stiffness. The most common forms of osteoarthritis of the back include spondylosis and spondylolisthesis, disc disease, and spinal stenosis. Musculoskeletal specialists can alleviate symptoms with exercise programs, medication, local therapies, and surgery if needed.

Table 8: Disorders, syndromes, and conditions associated with back or neck pain

Inflammatory

Autoimmune (e.g., rheumatoid arthritis, polymyalgia rheumatica)

Seronegative spondyloarthropathy (e.g., ankylosing spondylitis, psoriatic arthritis)

Related to inflammatory bowel disease

Crystal related
  (e.g., gout, pseudo-gout)

Metabolic/bone mineralization
  (e.g., osteoporosis, Paget's Syndrome, parathyroid disease)

Infections

Bone tumors (primary or metastatic)

Blood diseases
  (e.g., sickle cell anemia, leukemia)

Gastrointestinal

(GI) tract, genitourinary (kidney, bladder) or reproductive regions

Infiltrative or fibrosing
  (e.g., bone cyst, retroperitoneal fibrosis)

Neurologic
  (e.g., multiple sclerosis, nerve compression)

Psychiatric
  (e.g., psychogenic rheumatism, depression, malingering)

Fibromyalgia/ regional myofascial pain

Mechanical without osteoarthritis
  (e.g., trauma, strain, whiplash)

Fractures

Osteoarthritis with or without mechanical components

Generalized osteoarthritis (includes spondylosis, spondylolisthesis)

Herniated disc

Spinal stenosis

DISH (diffuse idiopathic skeletal hyperostosis)

Accelerated osteoarthritis (e.g., scoliosis)

Table 9: Radicular symptoms

Vertebrae	Pain distribution
C5	Neck to outer shoulder, arm
C6	Outer arm to thumb, index finger
C7	Outer arm to middle finger
C8	Inner arm to ring, little fingers
L4	Front of thigh to inner part of leg
L5	Outer side of leg to bottom of feet
S1	Lateral foot

13

The Lower Body

Undoings at Our Underpinnings

There's language in her eye, her cheek, her hip. Nay, her foot speaks, her wanton spirits look out. At every joint and motive of her body.

—William Shakespeare, (1564–1616)
Triolus and Cressida

The major joints involved in osteoarthritis of the lower extremity are in the hip, knee, ankle, and feet. Although the general principles of taking a history, performing a physical examination, and making a diagnosis are similar, each joint complex has its own unique pathology and characteristics. We'll cover these regions from top to bottom.

LET'S GET HIP

The hip joint represents a meeting of two of the largest bony structures of the body. A ball-and-socket joint four inches deep under the skin that cannot be felt, this joint connects the femur with the pelvis (Figure 21). The *femur* is the longest bone in the body and connects to the pelvis in a cavity known as the *acetabulum*, formed by the fusion of three pelvic bones: the ilium, ischium, and pubis. The joint is extremely stable. Anchored by strong ligaments and bursae, the femoral head is two thirds of a perfect sphere, 40% of which is enclosed by the acetabulum. The joint usually glides easily; its lubricating fluid and structure makes it several

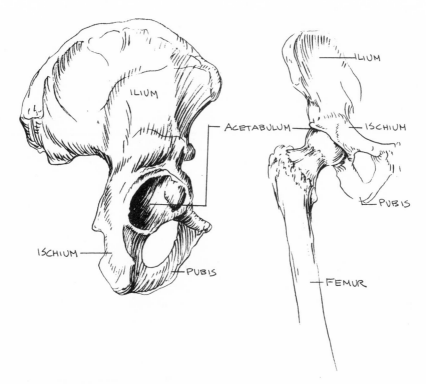

FIG. 21A *The hip joint*

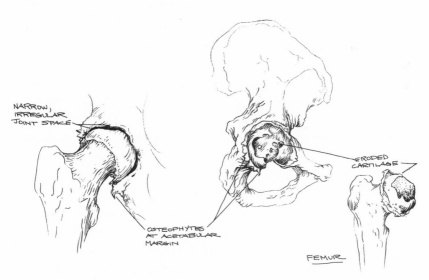

FIG. 21B *Osteoarthritis of the hip*

times more slippery than ice. The stability of this joint is reinforced by the deep insertion of the femur, strong fibrous capsules, and three groups of extremely strong muscles. Flexor muscles (such as the iliopsoas) allow us to bend; extensors (e.g., the gluteus maximus) promote straightening and are very bulky; and abductors (like the gluteus medius) prevent lurching. Also, three small muscles adduct the hip, allowing it to turn inward. All told, the hip joint lets us stand erect and permits walking, running, squatting, and dancing.

My hip hurts!

The most common symptom in this region is pain. Pain can come from many sources, some of which have nothing to do with the hip. For example, pain in the pelvic or reproductive areas and from certain abdominal conditions can present as hip discomfort. This is known as *referred pain*. Since nerves emanating from the lumbar spine (such as the sciatic nerve) traverse the hip region, low back and sacroiliac problems are often thought by patients to be hip-related. Similarly, degenerative conditions in the knee can produce differences in leg length and difficulty walking, which is incorrectly perceived as coming from the hip.

The most common condition related to the hip area is a *bursitis*. The fluid in the bursae frequently become inflamed or irritated as a consequence of poor body mechanics, osteoarthritis of the hip or lower spine, trauma, and athletic endeavors. (The principal hip bursae are shown in Figure 22.) *Trochanteric bursitis* affects just about everybody at some point, and produces pain at the side of the pelvis. Pain in the center of the buttocks is far more commonly due to an *ischial bursitis* or *iliopsoas bursitis* than from sciatica or osteoarthritis. The former, known as "weaver's bottom," is made worse by sitting all day. Iliopsoas bursitis pain starts in the buttocks and spreads to the groin area. Also, fibromyalgia tender points tend to overly these bursae. Sometimes patients complain of numbness in the upper leg and trochanteric area. This is due to compression of a superficial nerve (the lateral femoral cutaneous nerve) and is known as *meralgia paresthetica*. Meralgia tends to occur in patients who wear tight belts, corsets, or other garments. Muscles are attached to bones by tendons, and *tendinitis* of the abductor or adductor muscle groups, among others, are common as well. Other conditions should be considered when a patient complains of hip pain: inflammatory processes (such as rheumatoid arthritis), infection, tumors,

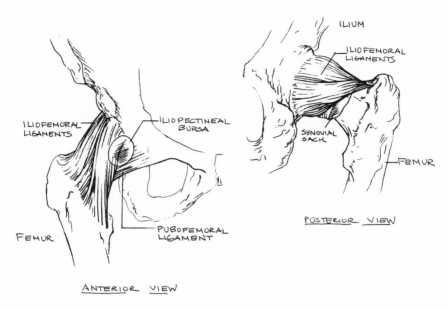

FIG. 22 *Hip bursae and ligaments*

traumatic injuries, and metabolic disorders (such as Paget's syndrome or osteoporosis).

The hip examination

When your doctor examines your hip, there are various things to assess. Are there any postural abnormalities? Are the leg lengths equal, or do there appear to be any contractures (inability to straighten a leg)? Your stance and gait is observed as you walk across the room. With pain, the body tilts towards the involved hip and appears to limp. Trying not to bear weight on the painful area produces an *antalgic gait* or waddle, which resembles a marionette's stride. At this point the hip and adjacent areas are palpated. Is the pain referred from the spine or abdomen? Is it the hip joint or a bursa or tendon that is the focus of discomfort? Next, the hip is manipulated through its range of motions. Are there decreases in its range of activities? Muscle strength is assessed by applying resistance to the flexors, extensors, abductors, and adductors. If necessary, similar maneuvers are repeated with the patient in a prone position.

Osteoarthritis of the hip

Karen was 70 years old when she saw Dr. Ling because her left knee hurt. The knee examination and her X-rays were normal. When Tylenol and Naprosyn failed to help, Karen was referred to an orthopedist. Dr. Jessup found marked decreased range of motion in the left hip. Karen walked with her toes turned out and the right leg was an inch longer than the left. Radiographic studies showed that the problem was in the hip and not the knee. Karen had advanced left hip osteoarthritis. Since she was starting to develop early knee flexion contractures and quadriceps weakness (which could end up putting her in a wheelchair), a hip replacement was scheduled.

Once tendonitis, bursitis, fibromyalgia, or disc problems are considered and ruled out, a diagnosis of osteoarthritis of the hip can be made. At least 5% of the United States population over the age of 55 has symptomatic hip arthritis. Suggested by decreased range of motion, its diagnosis is confirmed by a plain X-ray. Over time the joint space narrows: superiolaterally in 60%, of patients medial (towards the middle) in 25% and concentrically in 15%. Osteophytes form at the edges. In the early stages, pain is intermittent, focal, and associated with around a half hour of stiffness in the morning. The cartilage begins to disintegrate and rotation diminishes, and the pain increases in intensity. Ultimately, it becomes hard to walk, and pain occurs even at rest. Deformities and altered gait patterns, along with muscle weakness, become obvious.

Mild hip osteoarthritis is managed with weight loss, acetaminophen, nonsteroidal anti-inflammatory drugs, icing the area before activity, quadriceps strengthening exercises, and rest. Associated bursitis or tendonitis additionally responds to local corticosteroid injections. Each year, 100,000 Americans undergo the ultimate therapy: a hip replacement (described in further detail in chapter 20).

THE KNEE

As the largest joint in the body, the knee consists of three articulations, with one common articular cavity. The *patellofemoral, lateral,* and *medial tibial femoral condyles,* form a large diarthroidal joint (Figure 23). Supported by ligaments, muscles, and bursae, the knee folds on itself,

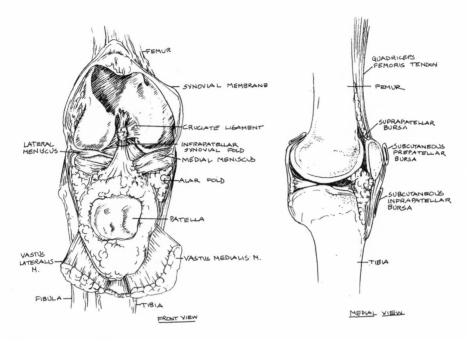

FIG. 23   *The knee joint*

bears two to three times your body weight with activity, and locks with extension. The knee has several unique features. A small sesamoid bone, the *patella* or knee cap, fits into a groove at the end of the femur and lies in the quadriceps tendon. It increases efficiency of the large *quadriceps* muscle. The quadriceps consists of four muscles behind the upper leg which extend, straighten, and allow bending of the knee. In front of them are three *hamstring* muscles. Originating at the knee and inserting in the ankle region is the calf muscle, or *gastrocnemius.*

The knee has a group of supporting structures (Figure 24). Ligaments, attaching bone to bone, stabilize the knee. Medial and lateral stability is provided by the *medial* and *lateral cruciate ligaments*. The *anterior* and *posterior cruciate ligaments* give rotation support and stabilize the knee as well. The *meniscus* consists of thick cartilage covering the surface of the tibia, which acts as a shock absorber.

Examining and imaging the knee

Where does the knee hurt? What makes it more or less painful? Is it hard to walk? Are you stiff or tender, and do you sense swelling or full-

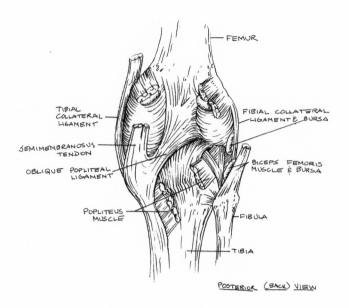

FIG. 24A *Supporting structures of the knee, posterior view*

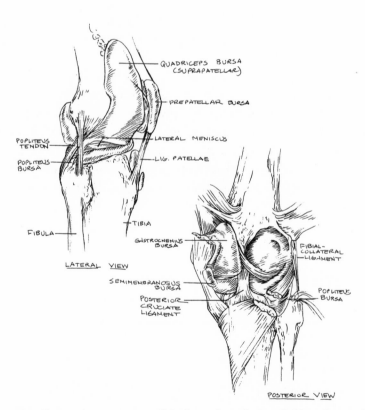

FIG. 24B *Supporting structures of the knee, lateral view (left) and posterior view (right)*

ness in the knee? Does the knee lock, or buckle? Do you or lose your balance or feel like you could fall? Does the pain come from the hip or go to the ankle? These are the initial questions your doctor should ask upon examination.

The knee is first inspected with the patient standing. Is there any postural deformity? Does the patient appear to be knock-kneed or bow-legged? Are there obvious leg length differences, or atrophy on one or both sides? Next, the knee is palpated. Is it tender, red, or warm, as in pseudo-gout or gout? Could the knee be swollen with fluid? (The knee has the largest synovial capsule in the body and forms extra fluid more often than any other joint; this can represent inflammation, infection, trauma, or advanced osteoarthritis.) Does the knee make sounds when it is moved? If so, this suggests ligament or tendon irritation or an internal derangement in the bony structure of the knee. The knee can be flexed (with the help of the hamstrings), extended (with the help of the quadriceps), or rotated (with support provided by the menisci and the medial, collateral and cruciate ligaments). The patient is often asked to walk, and pulses, reflexes, and lower extremity muscle strength are evaluated.

X-rays of the knee may be necessary to confirm clinical suspicions. Degenerative changes are represented by joint-space narrowing. Frequently, this narrowing is observed on one side. Medial narrowing (seen in 75% of patients with knee osteoarthritis) can create a knock-kneed appearance, while lateral narrowing (observed in 26% of knee osteoarthritis cases) is associated with a Charlie Chaplin-like gait. Almost half of patients with knee osteoarthritis have patello-femoral joint changes on X-rays. *Chondrocalcinosis,* or calcification of the cartilage, is more commonly seen in the knee than in any other joint. Some patients develop attacks of pseudo-gout, while others simply have osteoarthritis. Osteophyte formation at the joint or patellar margins is common with wear and tear and increasing age. X-rays can also demonstrate avascular necrosis, erosions (as in rheumatoid arthritis), osteochondromatosis (extra bones in the joint, known as "joint mice"), tumors, fractures, or infected bone. Since the ligaments, tendons, bursae, and menisci cannot be visualized on a regular X-ray, your doctor may also order MRI scan of the knee. More MRIs are performed on the knee than almost any other joint: they are used to diagnose meniscal tears, ligament ruptures, or inflammation of the knee joint and surrounding bursae, ligaments, tendons, and menisci; identify sacs of fluid; and often allow an orthopedist to ascertain if surgical or medical therapy is best for the patient. It is also the only study that can diagnose plica and chondromalacia patella (discussed in the next section). An ultrasound of the lower knee area may help your doctor determine if you have a ruptured Baker's cyst (the popliteal bursa) as opposed to phlebitis (inflammation of veins). If the problem is particularly difficult to pinpoint, a radiologist may inject dye into the knee joint and have you walk around. An *arthrogram*, (commonly performed in the days before MRI) can sometimes give doctors a definitive diagnosis if the MRI findings are not helpful.

Associated knee conditions

A variety of conditions are commonly seen when osteoarthritis is present in the knee. Most of them tend to be mechanical, or related to abnormal stresses placed on certain locations around the knee. Several types of bursitis are often mistaken for osteoarthritis of the knee. *Anserine bursitis* is a condition frequently in those who are overweight and sometimes co-exists with *adiposa dolorosa*, or painful fat pads around the knee. This bursa lies two inches below the knee joint on the medial side (Figure 25). Patients experience discomfort on climbing stairs, and the bursa is usually quite tender to touch. While rest, stretching and anti-inflammatory regimens are helpful, excellent results can also be obtained from a local injection of a corticosteroid/anesthetic combination into the bursa. The *popliteal bursa* lies behind the knee near the gastrocnemius. Vigorous contraction of the quadriceps forces fluid into this bursa when we walk. If the synorial lining is inflamed, the fluid forced into it cannot get out. Known as a "ball-valve" effect, the popliteal bursa can swell up and become a *Baker's cyst*, which can present as a painful huge balloon in the back of the leg. On occasion it pops, sending joint fluid down inside of the leg, which becomes very swollen and painful. Some doctors mistake a ruptured Baker's cyst for acute phlebitis. Fortunately, ultrasound evaluations quickly provide the definitive diagnosis. A Baker's cyst can be drained, injected, or even removed before it ruptures. Another condition, historically known as "housemaid's knee," a *prepatellar bursitis* is frequently found in those who spend a lot of time on their knees at work. Located in front of the kneecap, this painful condition is treated with preventive strategies, anti-inflammatory therapies, and local injections.

The knee is uniquely lined with *plica*. These linings can produce a lancinating, snapping, locking, or clicking sensation. Resembling a bow-

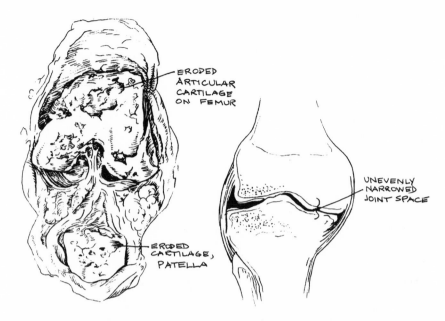

FIG. 25   *Osteoarthritis of the knee*

string, plica act as stretching scars and can become especially trouble-some after arthroscopy. Chronic inflammation and osteoarthritic changes are associated with plica-related symptoms. A variety of tendons can become inflamed in patients with knee osteoarthritis. One of the more common forms is *popliteal tendinitis*, also known as "jumper's knee." Chronic changes can produce calcification of ligaments, such as that found in diffuse idiopathic skeletal hyperostosis or DISH (chapter 12), or in *Pellegrini-Stieda syndrome*, where pain is produced by calcification of the medial collateral ligament in the knee.

Osteoarthritis of the knee

Celeste's right knee started to bow outward. At first it didn't hurt, but the outer area of the knee finally started to ache. When it became harder to walk because the left knee remained straight, she saw her family doctor. X-rays were consistent with lateral joint space narrowing with bone spurs and eburnation. Celeste was prescribed Advil to use as needed, a heel lift to wear in her shoe, and an exercise program. She is much better now, but her orthopedist has told her that a knee replacement may be in her future.

The onset of knee osteoarthritis can be accelerated in athletes and following injuries, but in otherwise healthy people doesn't usually appear until after the age of 50. Twenty percent of Americans over the age of 55 have symptomatic knee osteoarthritis. Medial or lateral asymmetrical narrowing of the joint from cartilage degeneration produces a malalignment of associated supporting structures, resulting in joint pain or an abnormal gait. Fraying and fibrillation of the cartilage ultimately lead to pseudo-gout calcium pyrophosphate crystals in the joint, loose bodies of bone, and a sense of buckling, locking, and contractures. The most common symptoms of knee osteoarthritis are pain and stiffness. Patients may not be aware of postural or gait abnormalities. Joint crystals are associated with acute pain, swelling, and tenderness. Cruciate ligaments, tendons, and meniscal degeneration are frequently found alongside degenerative changes in the knee.

Weight loss, exercise, shock-absorbing footwear, and other devices can help osteoarthritis of the knee. From a medication standpoint, if acetaminophen is not helpful, then aspirin, ibuprofen, or selective cox-2 anti-inflammatory regimens usually provide some relief. Corticosteroid injections (with or without a joint fluid aspiration) can lead to dramatic improvements. When injections fail or only give a few days of relief, doctors usually order an MRI scan to look for internal derangements in the knee that might require arthroscopic intervention. Torn menisci and ruptured cruciates can be repaired rather effectively in young and middle-aged patients. When bone-on-bone is seen on a knee X-ray, indicating the complete destruction of joint cartilage, a knee replacement may be necessary. Some doctors try *viscosupplementation,* or injection with hyaluronic acid derivatives, to buy a little more time or prevent surgery. Arthroscopic and surgical interventions are discussed in further detail in chapters 19 and 20.

A form of osteoarthritis unique to the patella or kneecap is known as *chrondromalacia patella.* Diagnosed with an MRI and treated optimally with arthroscopic patellar "shaving," this condition represents a softening and degeneration of the cartilage lining the patella. It produces pain in the front of the knee and the patello-femoral ligament. Patients with chrondromalacia patella have pain walking up and down stairs. Cases of mild to moderate severity are managed with quadriceps strengthening exercises, hamstring stretching, and nonsteroidal anti-inflammatory agents.

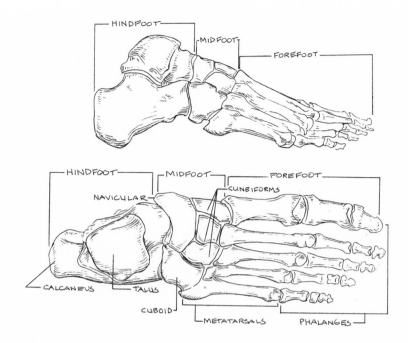

FIG. 26A   *Bones of the foot and ankle*

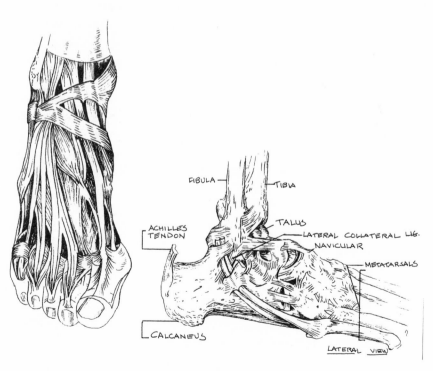

FIG. 26B   *Supporting structures of the foot and ankle*

GETTING OUR FEET WET

Our two feet somehow manage to support most of our body weight. This triumph of engineering biomechanics is performed by 26 bones, two arches, and numerous tendons, ligaments, and fascial sheaths. Acting as shock absorbers, our feet sustain an impact force of 63 tons per mile. Osteoarthritis of the feet is present in half of the population by the age of 75, which is a relatively low percentage considering the pounding these areas receive. Let's look at how the feet and ankle are constructed, and then we'll review how osteoarthritis affects these areas.

The foot and ankle are divided anatomically into three regions: the hindfoot, midfoot and forefoot. The first represents the ankle area. This hinge joint consists of the tibia and fibular attachments to the *talus* (heel bone) and *calcaneus* (ankle bone). Ankle articulations principally permit up and down motions (plantar and dorsiflexion), but no real rotation. The *Achilles tendon* is located in the hindfoot. It is the largest tendon in the body, originating in the lower calf and inserting into the heel. The hindfoot becomes the midfoot at the end of the calcaneous bone. Here five tarsal bones (the navicular, cuboid, and three cuneiforms) act as ball bearings and permit the rolling motions associated with walking. This includes the *subtalar joint*. The midfoot is supported by two arches (longitudinal and transverse), which function as "springs" in that they flatten when loaded and spring back when released. Children have flat feet, and arches develop with time. The forefoot consists of five rays (the toes), which, except for the great toe, have four bones each. The great toe has three bones. Forming a ball-and-socket joint, they are known as *metatarsals* and *phalanges* (proximal, middle, and distal).

The foot and ankle examination

The most common foot and ankle symptom is pain. Complaints of foot and ankle discomfort often have nothing to do with the foot or ankle, per se. As part of a physical examination, poor circulation to the legs, nerve injuries to the spine, skin ulcers or sores, leg length discrepancies, scoliosis, knee deformities, and any metabolic disorders need to be ruled out. This also includes assessing pulses or reflexes, and performing blood tests.

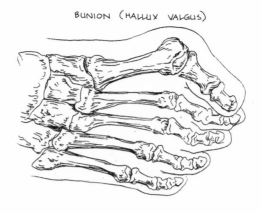

BUNION (HALLUX VALGUS)

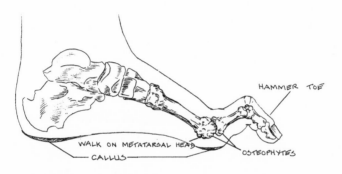

HAMMER TOE

WALK ON METATARSAL HEAD

CALLUS

OSTEOPHYTES

FIG. 27   *Osteoarthritis of the feet*

The most common direct causes of foot pain relate to ill-fitting shoes, minor injuries, or simply normal wear and tear. If it is believed that pain in the foot or ankle derives from local abnormalities, the first thing your doctor usually does is closely inspect the foot and ankle. Is there any obvious swelling or deformity? Can a bunion or hammer toe be identified? Are the arches absent (causing flat feet) or too high (as in *pes cavis*, or claw foot)? Do the soles of the feet show calluses? Next, the feet and ankle are felt. Is there warmth or tenderness? Does touching the Achilles tendon produce pain? Is the area of tenderness red or inflamed? The toes are squeezed to screen for neuromas or metatarsalgia. The patient may be asked to stand. Do the heels pronate (evert and abduct) or supinate (invert with abduction)? Does the pain depend on what position is assumed? Can the patient walk on the toes or heels? A gait analysis may also be performed. Sixty percent of the walking action is spent in a "stance" phase, where our feet are on the floor, and 40% in a "swing" phase consisting of acceleration, midswing, and deceleration. Flat feet, tight hamstrings (demonstrated by flexion contracture of a knee), and hip disease can be suggested by watching how we walk. Finally, the joints are "ranged" or moved about. Inability to dorsiflex the ankle at 20 degrees or plantar flex it more than 45 degrees suggests arthritic damage, tight ligaments, or damaged tendons. Increased range of motion may be found with a ligament rupture. The subtalar (talo-calcaneal) joint should invert to about 30 degrees and evert 20 degrees. Finally, the toes are evaluated. Where does it hurt and where are deformities? Has the great toe lost its ability to be flexed (*hallux rigidus*)? Looking at the kind of footwear being worn often provides the examiner with useful information. For example, high-heeled shoes suggest that the Achilles tendon might be irritated or inflamed, while those who prefer tennis shoes a half size too big frequently have metatarsal joint arthritis.

Blood tests may be ordered to screen for gout (suggested by inflammation of the great toe), rheumatoid arthritis (resulting in metatarsalgias or painful metatarsal joints), diabetes (which can cause numb toes), or other conditions. X-rays of the feet and ankle can identify osteoarthritis, rheumatoid arthritis, gout, stress fractures, and osteoporosis. CT scans or MRIs may be ordered, though this is done infrequently; CT provides very good images of the hindfoot, fibrous tissue, and cartilage, and MRI scans are generally ordered to confirm the presence of questionable stress fractures, infections, or tendon ruptures.

Conditions associated with osteoarthritis of the ankle or feet

Lynn wore stylish footwear for many years. Cramming her feet into narrow shoes with high heels began to take its toll. Her toes starting curling up, like a hammer, and the great toe began turning out. The same thing had happened to her mother. Lynn's podiatrist diagnosed her has having osteoarthritis and a bunion. Lynn was prescribed Celebrex, had her calluses shaved, and was advised to purchase an in-depth shoe. Although her feet don't look great, Lynn is no longer in pain and is anxious to avoid surgery.

Below the knee, osteoarthritis most frequently affects the first meta-tarsal-phalangeal (MTP) joint, followed by the subtalar joint and the ankle.

Degenerative changes of these joints alter body mechanics by putting stresses on supporting structures. All of the conditions discussed below are frequently found in patients with osteoarthritis of the feet and ankle.

Deformities due to osteoarthritis in the feet are common. The most common degenerative change is a *hallux valgus*, or bunion. Here the first MTP joint is malaligned, which causes medial bowing. Seen most often in women, hallux valgus has a strong genetic predisposition. It alters the alignment of adjacent toes, often producing a hammertoe effect, where they curl up like a claw: the interphalangeal joint is flexed, with the tip pointed downward. Bunions are managed by wearing loose-fitting shoes or sandals, or toe pads; they may be treated with nonsteroidal anti-inflammatory agents, orthotics, local corticosteroid injections, and surgery if needed. Hammer toe therapy involves manipulation, splinting, and using felt pads. Symptoms are rarely serious enough to require surgery. If the great toe cannot be flexed, the condition *hallux rigidus* is present. Also caused by osteoarthritis, patients are unable to press off their toes, and their feet turn out when they walk. Managed with mobilizers, stretching, rocker bar soles, and special shoes, treatment may involve nonsteroidal anti-inflammatory drugs or surgery. Some patients may need to use walkers, canes, or crutches.

Various *mechanical changes* can alter our feet over time. All children have flat feet, but with age the transverse and longitudinal arches mature and allow improved gait. Although some people with flat feet or claw feet (with a very high medial arch) never have symptoms, arch-related problems accelerate osteoarthritis. Very high arches produce calluses on the bottom of the feet. Flat feet put abnormal stresses throughout the supporting structures and bones of the feet, causing problems such as a very tight Achilles tendon or inflammation of the plantar fascia. Changes in mechanical stresses of the feet also produce a forefoot varus (inverted) or forefoot valgus (everted) appearance.

Chronic rheumatoid inflammation, foot strain, everted feet, trauma, osteoarthritis with hallux valgus, flat feet, and poor footwear can all create an environment where the ends of the metatarsal bones point downward, causing the major stress to fall on the metatarsal heads or balls of the feet. Since this part of the body handles the bulk of our downward weight, *metatarsalgia*, or painful metatarsals, is quite common. Metatarsal bars on the bottom of shoes or pads within shoes help shift weight off these bones, as does an in-depth shoe.

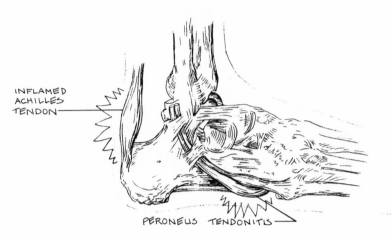

INFLAMED
ACHILLES
TENDON

PERONEUS   TENDONITIS

FIG. 28   *Example of foot tendonitis*

Tendinitis and bursitis are also common. Inflammation of the *Achilles tendon* can be induced by trauma, overactivity, ill-fitting shoes (especially if they have a stiff heel counter), and osteoarthritis of the ankle. The tendon may become tender and swollen. Managed by heel lifts and footwear modifications, and treatment with nonsteroidal anti-inflammatory drugs, the tendon generally should *not* be injected with corticosteroids. The most common cause of rupture of this tendon is from local injections, which, if attempted, needs to be done by a physician expert in dealing with this problem. *Retrocalcaneal bursitis* (subachilles bursitis) produces inflammation of the back of the heel and is frequently seen with Achilles tendinitis. Tendons going around the malleolus (a hammer-like prominence on either side of the ankle bone) frequently become inflamed. *Peroneal tendinitis* is lateral, while *posterial tibial tendinitis* is medial. Local injections are usually helpful.

Compressive nerve conditions are sometimes diagnosed when patients sometimes complain of pain, burning, or numbness at their metatarsals between the third and fourth toes. Seen primarily in middle-aged women, this represents entrapment of interdigital nerves and is known as *Morton's neuroma*. Local injections and metatarsalgia therapies usually relieve the discomfort. Surgical excision is also curative, but rarely needed. Like its carpal tunnel counterpart in the wrist, swelling and inflammation at the ankle and occasionally severe osteoarthritis of the joint lead to compression at the posterior tibial tendon. This nerve entrapment (termed *tarsal tunnel syndrome*) leads to numbness, burning, and tingling in the medial malleolus and leading to the foot. Local injections, and anti-inflammatory therapies are the treatments of choice.

Heel spurs can occur when a thick layer of connective tissue stretches from the heel bone to the toes on the underside of the foot. Known as the *plantar fascia,* this tissue becomes painful in some patients with flat feet and overuse syndromes. X-rays of the bottom of the heel sometimes show spurring. This is present in nearly 16% of patients with plantar fasciitis and may or may not cause symptoms. The discomfort is manifested as a burning and aching sensation, especially in the morning when walking is first attempted. Heel cord stretching, nonsteroidal anti-inflammatory therapies, and local injections can be beneficial.

SUMMARY

Osteoarthritis in the lower body can manifest itself in the hip, the knees, or the feet and ankles. Hip pain can be caused by problems in the hip, back, or knee. In the knee, the plica, menisci, and collateral ligaments play a role; while in the feet, footwear and gait biomechanics are especially important.

Part v

THE MANAGEMENT OF OSTEOARTHRITIS

The art of medicine is to follow Nature, to imitate and assist her in the cure of diseases.

—Thomas Reid,
Inquiry into the Human Mind
on the Principles of Common Sense (1785)

If we thought treating osteoarthritis was easy, it would not involve eleven chapters of discussion. If there were a satisfactory treatment, we would not need so much room to relate various therapies. You may be surprised to learn that a lot of the factors involved in managing osteoarthritis are things you can do for yourself. Chapter 14 reviews psychosocial support; chapter 15, how to create an optimal home and work environment which decreases pain; and chapter 16 discusses exercises to improve osteoarthritis. Most osteoarthritis patients do, however, also benefit from medications. After discussing how these medicines are tested (chapter 17), those which clearly work are reviewed in chapters 18 and 19, and those which might, in chapter 22. Surgical options are delineated in chapter 21, and the role of non-rheumatologists and non-orthopedists is discussed in chapter 23. Sometimes osteoarthritis sufferers are children, or pregnant women, or people in so much pain that special considerations apply. Individuals interested in these issues are referred to chapters 20 and 24.

14

You Can Conquer Osteoarthritis

A thousand ills require a thousand cures.
—Ovid, *A Love's Cure*, A.D. 8

You've been diagnosed with osteoarthritis. It's clear that it is a chronic condition that won't simply go away. You know that going to the doctor is important, taking medicine may be advisable, and even surgery might be required. However, there is more you can do to deal with osteoarthritis. The good news is that there are many approaches which enable patients to help themselves. It's possible to improve arthritis pain, function, and performance without ever going to the doctor. In the next three chapters, some self-help approaches and physical measures will be reviewed.

WHY IS OSTEOARTHRITIS SO SPECIAL?

Osteoarthritis differs from many other disorders. In most patients with the disease, it is present for a third of a lifetime, and pain is its principal bothersome feature. All too often, when the new osteoarthritis sufferer sees a doctor, they are told to learn to live with it. Unfortunately, they are rarely told *how* to do this. After all, osteoarthritis is disruptive. It requires confronting new issues of medical care and accommodating to life changes. While your doctor thinks of osteoarthritis in the mind-set of what is anatomically wrong or functionally deficient, patients have a different set of thoughts: Why do I feel bad? How much do I know

119

about the disease? What behaviors best solve my problems? How do I manage my frustrations and fears?

There is a lot more to osteoarthritis than joint pain. For example, individuals with depression who happen to have osteoarthritis use disproportionately high levels of health care services provided by arthritis specialists compared to those with osteoarthritis alone. Tricyclic antidepressants are medicines which help diminish depression. Although they have absolutely no effect upon osteoarthritis, the use of these agents is associated with less arthritis pain. On the other hand, senior citizens are notoriously stubborn and do everything they can to remain self-reliant. They are tremendous underutilizers of mental health services.

What's the best way to handle these problems? First, see your doctor. Let them assess your joints and determine what's wrong anatomically and functionally. Second, your doctor needs to assess you—as a person. What is the impact and severity of your pain? What is your level of distress or handicap? What other medical problems are you having? How does this impact upon your quality of life? Do you have a social support system? How much do you know about arthritis? Once this is factored into the equation, the correct management direction can be formulated. This includes educating you about osteoarthritis, controlling pain, optimizing function, and decreasing any handicaps.

HONE YOUR COPING SKILLS

Life may deal us bad hands at times, but failing to confront unpleasant realities only makes things worse. Osteoarthritis produces changes in our lives via three paths. First, it alters our daily activities, including working, household chores, and recreational endeavors. Second, it produces new thought patterns. How does this affect us and others? How does it influence the future? Finally, osteoarthritis can produce feelings of anxiety, anger, and depression.

Coping is the vehicle we use to confront these changes. There are many ways to cope, and it's important to choose the one which serves your best interests. An osteoarthritis sufferer may initially feel confrontational, employ distancing with loved ones, or attempt to avoid the issue altogether, hoping it will just go away. Self-control and planned problem solving will allow positively focused reappraisals of what you are doing with your life. It often helps to identify the specific osteoarthritis problem (e.g., "I can't completely extend my knee"). Once the source has been pinpointed, think about how the problem affects your daily activities. What are the best ways to solve the problem? What resources are available to you? Would it be helpful to seek social support, such as applying for disability or a meals-on-wheels program? Approach your problem positively, and you can overcome the deficit.

If your ability to perform daily activities is overwhelmed by an osteoarthritic impairment, don't get angry. Accept the new playing field. Learn to delegate. Prioritize what needs to be done and don't get upset if you cannot do it all. Above all, communicate. Seek all the information necessary to solve a problem. Never be shy about verbalizing your feelings. Listen to the concerns of others—they may be trying to help. Have a positive attitude and compensate for whatever functional deficit is problematic.

LIFE CHANGES DUE TO OSTEOARTHRITIS: DO YOU HURT BECAUSE YOU'RE DEPRESSED OR IS IT THE OTHER WAY AROUND?

Compared to other forms of arthritis, most osteoarthritis patients cope rather well. A summary of studies shows that depression is prominent in 50% of patients with fibromyalgia, 42% with rheumatoid arthritis, 40% with systemic lupus, and 31% with ankylosing spondylitis—but only 14% with osteoarthritis. However, if osteoarthritis of the knee, neck, or hip are the prominent complaint, the percentage rises to 20. What is depression? Historically described as "helplessness and hopelessness," it contains many facets. A disorder of mood, some of its more obvious effects are sadness, irritability, and excessive worrying. It can also lead to a lack of interest in normal activities, loss of ability to concentrate, low self-esteem, social withdrawal or dependency, and changes in bodily functions (such as poor sleep, loss of sexual drive, fatigue, and pain). The strongest predictors of depression among osteoarthritis patients are pain, anxiety, low self-esteem and functional impairment.

How does depression influence osteoarthritis? If we lose interest in our friends, don't feel like eating, ignore our personal care, have no libido, can't sleep, argue with everybody, and can't think clearly, it can be difficult to enjoy living. This further lowers our self-image, saps our energy, and worsens mood swings. Depression also leads to fear or panic concerning illness. How is my body going to change? Will I become dependent upon others? Uncertainty and frustration take over when it becomes hard to rely on oneself, and anger is a natural response. Don't others know that I hurt? Why can't you be more helpful? These are typical reactions. Unfortunately, it leads to a vicious cycle which makes things worse.

GETTING OUT THE DOLDRUMS: MIND-SETS THAT HELP

Al's right hip hurt. He had just retired from a fulfilling, 40-year optometry practice, had always been in great health, and the timing could not have been worse. His wife, Rita, was diagnosed with breast cancer and their only daughter's employer sold his business, so she was transferred to Dallas. Al found it hard to sleep and started becoming quick to anger, and never felt like going out. Dr. Jones took X-rays and diagnosed Al as having moderately severe hip osteoarthritis. He was told to take two Aleve twice a day whenever the pain bothered him. Despite this, Al only modestly improved and still complained of significant hip discomfort. Physical therapy was prescribed, and a more detailed musculoskeletal evaluation by the therapist revealed significant muscular tension in the upper back, neck, and buttocks area. Elavil, an antidepressant with muscle relaxing properties, was added to the regimen along with counseling. Al began to sleep better and kept to his exercise regimen. He is experiencing less hip pain and seems to be turning the corner.

Depression is a reaction to pain and emotional stress in individuals whose coping skills are overwhelmed. There are many constructive approaches towards overcoming depression and other concerns associated with osteoarthritis. Let's see how this can be done.

First, take stock. What are your long-term goals? Decide what it is you want to accomplish. For example, if becoming more active is one of these goals, what are the best steps towards accomplishing this?

STRESS AND RELAXATION

Today's arthritis sufferer is often overcome by challenges of living in our fast-paced, advanced society. While certain forms of stress can be energizing and allow us to meet exciting challenges, other types can cause us to lose focus, become depressed, anxious, panicky, and make it difficult to think clearly. Pain and impairment due to osteoarthritis may further aggravate stressful situations. Relaxation rests our muscles and joints. It makes it harder to think about arthritis. This form of quiet time should take place in a comfortable environment. Wear loose-fitting clothes. Lay down or sit. Learn to deep-breathe. All sorts of devices reinforce relaxation. Guided imagery transports your mind to another time and place where good feelings and thoughts govern the psyche. Try to dissociate the painful part of the body from your mind. Distraction is very important. Pleasing sounds and activities (playing cards, reading a book, or prayer) make it difficult to think of your arthritis pain. Biofeedback and other modalities provided by therapists are reviewed in chapter 15.

GET A GOOD NIGHT'S SLEEP

Osteoarthritis patients often sleep poorly. A good night's sleep is important in order to repair the muscular microtrauma that occurs during the day, and also allows our body to make enough endorphins, which decrease pain. Daytime fatigue diminishes and our ability to concentrate improves. There are many rules of sleep hygiene that don't require taking a sleeping pill or seeing a doctor. Find a quiet bedroom with a comfortable bed and a firm mattress. Make sure the room is dark, your bed partner does not snore, and that pets sleep in another room. Use earplugs if necessary. Try not to nap during the day, and don't have caffeine or alcohol after mid-afternoon. Don't exercise in the evening. When you are getting ready for bed, create an environment which puts your mind in the sleep mode. Don't watch horror movies or read scary books. Play soft, pleasing music. Take a hot shower and relax your muscles. If you have osteoarthritis in the lower back, you might wish to place a pillow under the knees. This makes things worse if you have osteoarthritis in the knees; in that case, a pillow under the ankles is desirable. Discomfort at night from osteoarthritis of the cervical spine is best managed with a cervical pillow, which prevents hyperextension (thus leading to pain and spasm) of the neck. Patients with hip problems benefit from resting on their stomach occasionally because it helps prevent hip contractures.

A GOOD SEX LIFE IS IMPORTANT

I once had a patient who had osteoarthritis in her hip. After five years of visiting me several times a year, it was apparent that she had become irritable, moody, and depressed. It turned out that her partner refused to have sex after finding out about her arthritis. He was afraid of physically injuring her. It took her five years to confide this concern. Patients with hip osteoarthritis may have difficulty spreading their legs, but this does not preclude rear entry or other positions. Sex represents a form of intimacy and affection which provides pleasure, approval, and acceptance. Nearly all osteoarthritic deformities or impairments can be constructively worked with to allow continued sexual enjoyment. If this is a concern, be sure to verbalize it!

FEEL GOOD ABOUT YOURSELF

Just because you have osteoarthritis, this in no way lowers your self-worth or value to society. Helping others is a very rewarding, comforting feeling. Some arthritis sufferers advocate performing random acts of kindness. Have a phone buddy for support. Work promotes a sense of fulfillment and improves self-esteem. Even if you are disabled, retired, or limited in your ability to function, most people can volunteer and impart their wisdom and experience to others.

ENHANCE YOUR SOCIAL SUPPORT SYSTEM

Society has provided a variety of outlets to extend social support to the osteoarthritis sufferer. These outlets can be emotional (helping individuals develop feelings of belonging and being valued); informational (educating patients about osteoarthritis); and tangible (financial services and assistive devices). Counseling is available from physicians, psychologists, social workers, counselors, clergy, or role models. Though a small minority with osteoarthritis take advantage of this form of intervention, the potential benefits of psychosocial support towards treating depression, anxiety, and low self-esteem cannot be overemphasized. Several published studies have demonstrated that cognitive behavioral therapy (which involves relaxation techniques and training in improving one's self-worth) has favorable impact upon the course of osteoarthritis. The Arthritis Foundation sponsors self-help courses in the United States which are of tremendous informational value. These two-hour, six-session courses explain what osteoarthritis is, review the role of exercise and lifestyle adjustments, and review medical and surgical interventions. The success of patient education has been validated in numerous published studies.

FAMILY, FRIENDS, AND COMMUNITY

Your immediate family and friends can provide a wonderful support system. They can provide emotional support, create a safe and functional home, help get you up and around, transport you to work or to the doctor's office, and assist with rehabilitation after surgery. Not all of us are fortunate enough to have such as support system. Indeed, in dysfunctional families, additional sources of stress can make it harder to fight arthritis. Many people live alone and rely on friends and community support networks. If you have a specific support giver, try to include that individual in discussions with your doctor or other health professional. Its important to maintain social ties and friendships outside of the home, even if it's by telephone, fax, or e-mail. Isolation only compounds the ability to function independently and allows you to dwell on pain and decreased function. Can you shop for food or cook meals? Are they of adequate nutritional value? If you can't drive because of a bad hip, are there friends or family who can take you places, or is there adequate public transportation or taxi service?

Most communities have outreach programs that osteoarthritis patients are eligible for. The Arthritis Foundation also sponsors exercise classes. Local governments and agencies have recreational programs and extend additional social services. Voluntary health agencies and churches underwrite resources for emotional support, friendships, meals, transportation, and counseling.

DOCTOR-PATIENT RELATIONSHIPS

One of the most important decisions you have to make is who should be in charge of your musculoskeletal care. Depending upon circumstance, the doctor could be a physician (e.g., an orthopedist or rheumatologist), a podiatrist, osteopath, or chiropractor. Is your doctor qualified? Is he or she board-certified, academically affiliated, or have a research unit? Do you feel comfortable with them?

Patients often have complaints about their doctor. Make sure that you can ask questions whenever necessary. Instructions should be clear and concise. Access to a musculoskeletal specialist may be limited by health plans. Patients have told us that doctors often don't spend enough time with their patients, tell them to try one pill after another, never explain what they think or are doing, don't listen, and make patients feel uncomfortable. No qualified health care professional should ever get upset if you wish a second opinion. Mutual honesty and respect, a sense of understanding of lifestyles and limitations on both sides, and open lines of communication are vital.

The extent to which a doctor-patient relationship is effective can, in part, be measured by compliance. Evaluated by the extent to which a person's behavior (e.g., taking a prescribed medication, following or executing recommended lifestyle changes) coincides with medical health, adherence rates are alarming low with osteoarthritis. Among several published surveys, the adherence rates range from 16–84% for taking medicine as prescribed, 39–85% for making lifestyle or dietary adjustments, and 25–65% for wearing prescribed hand splints. Reasons for noncompliance include family factors (such as lack of knowledge about the disease, poor coping, dysfunctional family environment, lack of money, or low self-esteem); avoidance factors (such as a patient feeling too young to have the disease, or not believing that it is serious); and regimen factors (cost, complexity, or difficulty). Obviously, both doctors and patients have a long way to go.

SUMMARY

You have been diagnosed with osteoarthritis and want to know what can be done to help yourself. Examine your surroundings. What can't you do? How will this alter your lifestyle? How much pain are you in? Be introspective. How are you dealing with osteoarthritis? Is your reaction appropriate? What modifications can be made to solve the problems? Learn about the disease. Find a good doctor you can communicate with. In the next two chapters, we will review how to deal with pain, and describe physical measures which improve your ability to function.

15

Living Well with Osteoarthritis

Bodily exercises are to be done discretely; not to be taken evenly and alike by all men.

—Thomas à Kempis,
The Imitation of Christ (1426)

In the previous chapter, we learned how to help deal with osteoarthritis from an emotional standpoint and become educated about the disease. But before we talk about arthritis medications, we must turn to our environment. How do we get through the day? What should we eat? Is there a role for physical or occupational therapy? How does the weather affect arthritis? How can we make our home friendlier and enjoy our vacations? Exercises that allow improved functioning will be discussed in the next chapter.

WHAT SHOULD I EAT, AND IS IT IMPORTANT TO LOSE WEIGHT?

Is there a special diet for arthritis? After all, arthritis diets are a multi-million-dollar-a-year industry. Patients with rheumatoid arthritis are told to eat fish; those with gout are directed to avoid organ meats, rich meat gravies, and alcohol; and people with lupus should not eat alfalfa sprouts. Does any of this apply to osteoarthritis? Not really. Many patients with osteoarthritis of the lower extremity are overweight. Weight loss and exercise help ameliorate the symptoms and progression of hip, knee, ankle, and foot osteoarthritis. But is there any specific diet, or foods that should or should not be eaten? No. A well-balanced, healthy diet is all that is necessary. Some patients with osteoarthritis have difficulty cooking meals for themselves. Take-out dinners or meals-on-wheels programs might be helpful. Monitoring portions helps with weight loss issues. Assistive devices reviewed later in this chapter allows individuals with osteoarthritis to be more independent in their kitchen. Osteoarthritis patients whose activity is limited by their disease need less food, especially if they do not exercise. Also, depression related to osteoarthritis can result in overeating. Weight loss can decrease the odds for developing osteoarthritis; in one survey, a weight reduction of 11 pounds was found to cut the risk of developing osteoarthritis in half.

ARE MINERALS, VITAMINS, OR OTHER FOOD SUPPPLEMENTS USEFUL?

Osteoarthritis is associated with osteoporosis, and patients with lower bone density are at increased risk for developing osteoarthritis and having it progress. Characterized by the loss of calcium in bone and manifested ultimately by increased bony fractures, osteoporosis can be retarded and prevented by a variety of strategies. These include taking in at least one gram of calcium daily, along with two multivitamins. Two multivitamin tablets taken daily usually contain enough Vitamin D to optimize the absorption of calcium from the gastrointestinal tract. Table 10 (at the end of this chapter) lists foods and preparations which enable patients to take in enough calcium. See also Chapter 22, for more discussion of alternative therapies.

Some vitamins are antioxidants. Vitamins A, C, and E protect against oxidative damage to cells and tissues and are capable of favorably influencing biologic reactions that promote bone and collagen synthesis. Controlled trials using these vitamins for osteoarthritis are small-scale and inconclusive, but hold out the potential for benefit.

REHABILITATION: WHEN CAN I BENEFIT FROM OCCUPATIONAL OR PHYSICAL THERAPY?

Most of us aren't sure what occupational therapists or physical therapists do. Occupational therapy has little to do with "occupation" per se, and physical therapy provides a lot more than massage. (There's more on the educational background and qualifications for these professionals in chapter 22.). How can we tell if these are appropriate for you? The goals of any rehabilitation program need to be realistic, reasonable, precisely defined, and include preventive measures.

Occupational therapists evaluate the degree of articular involvement present, the amount of pain and joint stiffness you have, any deformities, and psychosocial needs, among others. They perform an ADL, or activities of daily living evaluation. This lets them know what you can and cannot do, what's difficult or painful, who helps get things done and your attitude towards it, and what you want to do. More specifically, for instance, can you comb your hair, grip a pen, or bend your fingers? They examine your ability to provide self-care, manage your home, perform at work, and participate in leisure activities.

Once an occupational therapy evaluation is completed, a therapeutic plan is implemented based on the principles of protecting the joints and conserving energy. Joint protection strategies include distributing stresses to larger joints; using joints in the best mechanical position, making available adaptive equipment and splinting when needed; and avoiding repetitive activities. For example, a patient may be directed to avoid twisting the hand, wrist, or thumb, or seat heights may be raised for those with lower extremity osteoarthritis. Energy conservation principles involve setting priorities so that you only perform absolutely necessary tasks when feeling ill, distributing tasks over time, allowing for rest periods, utilizing relaxation strategies by balancing periods of rest with periods of activity, allowing for leisure and spiritual enrichment in your lifestyle, and not entirely eliminating an activity but doing some of it. A patient might be instructed to get eight to ten hours of sleep at night, resting the joints with splints, or unload the joints by losing weight.

Occupational therapy's aim is oriented towards creating an efficiency that may not have been important before. Is the task necessary? If so, how can it be simplified, who should do it, and what's the best time of day or the best period of time to have it done? Can storage areas be better organized? Where can wheels and levers best be used? Wheels decrease lifting of trash cans and suitcases, while levers used as handles or attachments can greatly improve functioning at work or at home. When should enlarged handles be advised?

Physical therapists improve our level of function through exercise, facilitating transfers, and evaluating how we walk. Function is assessed by looking at levels of self-care, control over the bowel and bladder, mobility, the ability to communicate, and social contacts. They assess your disease stage, which joints are involved, the influence of body mechanics, your lifestyle, and motivations. Both physical and occupational therapists teach patients how to distribute a load over stronger joints in a larger surface area, how to use the body as leverage and avoid using the same joint position for prolonged periods of time, and promote good posture. For example, patients should stand up straight, tuck their stomachs in, contract their buttock muscles, wear comfortable shoes, sit in a straight-back chair, and have a desk high enough so that they don't hunch over.

ASSISTIVE DEVICES USED BY THERAPISTS AND OTHER REHABILITATION SPECIALISTS

Rehabilitation specialists are adept at advising which assistive devices should be used to allow optional functioning. A *splint* is a rigid or flexible appliance used to prevent motion of a joint, or for fixation of displaced or moveable parts. Usually employed for wrist or finger disease, the purpose is to maintain and enhance motion. Splints can decrease pain and inflammation, prevent or correct a deformity, and are helpful after an operation to maintain a position. Splints can be resting, functional or corrective and may be prefabricated or made by physical or occupational therapist to your specifications. Most are lightweight, plastic, and contain Velcro straps. *Collars* support the neck in patients with severe osteoarthritis and herniated discs. Lumbar *corsets, bands,* and *braces* can improve function and alleviate low back pain associated with disc disease.

Canes, crutches, or walkers assist ambulation. *Canes* are the simplest walking aid. They provide support and take pressure off the hips and knees. All canes should have a good rubber tip at the bottom. The tops can be straight like a T, curved like a candy cane, or round. Have your doctor check that adjustable canes are set at the correct height. *Crutches* are supported by the arm pits and require good shoulder function (with the exception of platform or forearm models). They provide more support than canes and are particularly useful after foot, ankle, or knee surgery in decreasing the load on these areas. *Walkers* can be folding, wheeled, rolling with a seat, or on a platform. They are most frequently employed after hip or back surgery and in patients with higher levels of impairment.

Shoe modifications or inserts are called *orthotics.* They can be fabricated (made of cork, leather, or plastic) at the recommendation of physicians, especially orthopedists, rheumatologists, and podiatrists. An orthotic can redistribute weight to a more normal pattern as we walk, reduce excessive pronation and knee pain, provide arch support for flat feet, act as a cushion and shock absorber, decrease pain from heel spurs, and support biomechanical malalignment. Metatarsal pads or bars redistribute weight. Molded shoes, in-depth shoes (large shoes which will allow for any deformities), or simply wearing a sneaker a half size too big may be needed.

Assistive devices recommended by occupational therapists promote personal hygiene by improving one's ability to bathe, dress, eat and transfer. This increases mobility and allows work, home, and school activities. Patients must learn to respect pain, balance work and rest, conserve energy, avoid positions of deformity, and use larger and stronger joints. This might mean using Velcro straps, shoes with wide toe areas, or long handled sponges in the bathtub. Hand osteoarthritis discomfort is minimized by wearing pullover sweaters to avoid difficulty in manipulating buttons. Flexible canes, held on the side opposite the affected side, improve hip pain; heel lifts decrease leg length discrepancies. Knee osteoarthritis is ameliorated by raised toilet seats and avoiding putting pillows under the knees while sleeping. More assistive devices are listed in Table 11, at the end of the chapter.

With the advent of prefabricated splints, braces, and supports, *taping* has become a type of lost art. Once applied to just about any part of the body, taping today is primarily used by trainers on athletic teams for sports injuries. An example of how taping helps knee osteoarthritis is in the management of patello-femoral syndrome. Taping the patello-femoral ligament in the lateral, neutral, or medial position decreases pain with kneeling, squatting, or climbing stairs.

Applied rehabilitation: Your home, car, and travel

How does all the above translate to your daily life? Let's look at your house. Is it adequately lit with easy-to-reach switches? Are the stones in your driveway level? Do the stairs have a banister? Are table and desk heights proper? Can items be carted around? Consider using a lazy Susan (circular shelves, so you don't have to reach), having electrical plugs and phone jacks at waist level, peg boards in the kitchen for your pots and pans, paper plates and utensils if it's difficult to wash dishes, and long handles. Labor-saving devices in the kitchen include mixers, microwave ovens, and electric can openers. Avoid putting things in high cupboards, write with felt marker pens, and don't write for long periods of time. Have somebody help you carry in the groceries and buy non-skid rugs.

When travelling in a car, make sure the vehicle has a good bucket seat and a wide angle mirror; keep knees higher than the hips, swing legs into the seat, and stop driving at least once an hour. Is the seat adjustable, and does it have armrests? Patients with low back pain may benefit from a lumbar seat, or support cushion (for example a Sacro-Ease-like accessory).

If you are on vacation, use nonpeak travel times, suitcases that roll, and pack lightly. Find a travel partner and get a good night's rest. It's important to get out and around. Don't isolate yourself!

IS THERE AN IDEAL CLIMATE FOR OSTEOARTHRITIS?

Most patients with osteoarthritis report that they feel more comfortable in warmer weather. In the winter, those living in colder climates should keep warm, use electric blankets as needed, and stay mobile. Osteoarthritis patients are also sensitive to changes in the barometer, and weather shifts from hot to cold or wet to dry are associated with increased stiffness or aching. This may worsen for a day or two when travelling to a different part of the country, and generally some time is necessary to adjust.

WHAT KIND OF HEAT IS BEST FOR MY JOINTS?

A feeling of warmth is welcome to many osteoarthritic joints. Heat decreases stiffness and pain, diminishes muscle spasms, and improves blood flow to joints. Heat can be applied to joints in several different ways. *Superficial heat* decreases intra-articular temperatures initially, and does not penetrate deeper joints such as the hip or knee. It may be applied using a hot pack, hydrocollator, or paraffin baths at forty-one to forty-five degrees centigrade. Patients with painful Hebreden's nodes in their fingers find that paraffin (a wax with mineral oil) is a soothing analgesic in the bath.

Deeper heat is less commonly applied, and more controversial. It delivers dry heat to patients with cancer, bleeding disorders, and marked inflammation. Short-wave diathermy, with or without electromagnetic pulses, can cover large areas through direct radiation but can also easily produce local burns. Ultrasound employs high-energy sound waves, which are helpful for pain relief and muscle spasms for short periods. Another form of deep heat, microwave, is no longer used to treat arthritis.

Moist heat is usually superior to *dry heat*. Water therapies benefit arthritis in general, since the buoyancy of water allows joints to move in positions they might not be able to assume under normal circumstances. Water therapy increases body temperature, and produces sweating and superficial dilation of blood vessels. It can increase the heart and respiratory rate while lowering blood pressure. Warm water immersion relaxes muscles, induces a sense of fatigue, and sedates sensory nerve endings.

ARE COLD APPLICATIONS OF ANY BENEFIT?

While most osteoarthritis patients feel better when they apply heat, cold applications help acute spasms and are useful for inflammatory complications such as pseudo-gout. Ideally, cold should decrease pain, swelling, inflammation, and spasm by reducing blood flow to an area and decreasing the release of histamine, a chemical that produces pain. It also lowers nerve velocity to a region and slows down the body's metabolism. The local constriction of blood supply is temporary and is followed by a rebound dilation of blood supply upon its discontinuation. Cold applications often increase joint pain in patients with Raynaud's phenomenon (a condition where one's fingers turn blue, and white in cold weather) and in heavy smokers. Cold packs, immersion, ice cube massage, or an evaporating spray such as ethyl chloride or fluorimethane are common methods of application.

MASSAGE

Massage, heat, and cold are the chief modalities utilized by physical therapists to alleviate pain. Massage involves several movements such as compression, striking, pounding, and kneading, all of which can produce musculoskeletal discomfort. Most osteoarthritis patients prefer gentle massage, often in concert with other treatments such as heat.

Massage applied to acupuncture points is called *acupressure.* There are no controlled studies documenting any precise benefits of massage for osteoarthritis, although it is known to be beneficial if associated muscles are in spasm.

LOCAL ELECTRICAL STIMULATION

The application of electrical pulses to painful areas is a mainstay of physical therapy. A variety of methods can deaden painful nerve signals to joints, which in turn raises the pain threshold of the patient. One of the most common is the *transcutaneous electrical nerve stimulation* (TENS) unit. These units can be used during a therapy session, and in more severe cases are worn by the patient, who can deliver a pulse when desired. High-frequency TENS stimulates sensory nerve endings, while low-frequency TENS stimulates the motor end plates of muscles. The therapeutic principle of TENS is that delivering low-level electrical impulses over the skin of an affected area overloads the nerve pathway, and thus overrides pain impulses. It also releases endorphins into the spinal cord, which decreases painful stimuli from type A and C fibers.

Some therapists concentrate on acupuncture points during electrical stimulation while other use "burst mode" or "inferential" methods (two simultaneous medium-frequency alternating currents) to decrease spasm and stiffness. TENS units should not be used in patients with pacemakers or use other electrical pumps or devices. Three well-controlled studies have shown that this treatment has modest beneficial effects in osteoarthritis.

Over the last few years there has been increased interest in *pulsed electromagnetic field* stimulation. Nerve stimulators have been used for years to promote bone formation after orthopedic procedures, and a few studies have suggested that it also modestly decreases osteoarthritis pain.

SUMMARY

There are many ways in which osteoarthritis patients can help themselves. In addition to a positive attitude and motivation, patients can improve their home environments to allow increased productivity and comfort with simple labor-and pain-saving devices and strategies. Calling upon a rehabilitation specialist, such as a physical or occupational therapist, further enhances the ability to enjoy activities of daily living by receiving instruction in principles of energy conservation and joint protection. Next, exercise programs which complement these efforts are reviewed.

Table 10: Calcium supplementation

Foods with high calcium content
(the average U.S. diet contains 600 mg a day)

Milk, 8 oz, 300 mg	Hard cheese, 1 oz, 200 mg
Ice cream, 1 cup, 176 mg	Oysters, ½ cup, raw, 113 mg
Broccoli, 1 cup, 136 mg	Sardines, canned, 3 oz, 372 mg
One large orange, 78 mg	Spinach, ½ cup, raw, 111 mg

Oral calium supplements, with examples of calcium products.
Never take in over 600 mg at a time. The body does not absorb more. Reserve some calcium for bedtime.

Calcium carbonate: OsCal, Tums, Titralac, Maalox, Mylanta
Calcium citrate: Citrical, caltrate
Calcium gluconate: Calcet
Calcium lactate: store brands

Vitamin D improves the absorption of calcium by the gastrointestinal tract.
The easiest way to get enough Vitamin D is by taking two multivitamins a day.

Table 11: Assistive Devices

General daily living
    Knob or faucet turners
    Key holders
    Loop or spring-loaded scissors

Ambulation assists
    Canes
    Crutches
    Walkers
    Orthotics

Mobility
   Corsets
   Bands
   Splints
   Braces
   Collars

Self-care: personal hygiene
   Long or enlarged brush or comb handles
   Toothbrush handles and pump toothpaste dispensors
   Enlarged razor handles
   Toilet tongs to hold paper or extend reach
   Long-handled sponge or brush
   Liquid soap with wall mounted dispensor
   Sponge or wash mitt

Self-care: dressing and eating
   Velcro closures rather than hooks
   Sewn-in loops for easy pull-up
   Long-handled shoehorn
   Two-handle glass holders
   Angled knife
   Extended straws
   Utensil handle grips

Transfers
   Elevated toilet seat and commode rails
   Tub rails or shower stools
   Chairs with arm supports
   Bed trapeze

Home management and activities
   Jar openers, utensils with large handles
   Electric food chopper, microwave
   Lightweight sweeper, long broom with attached dust pan
   Lightweight power tools
   Speakerphone

16

Exercises to Improve Osteoarthritis

Those who think they have not time for bodily exercise will sooner or later have to find time for illness.
—Edward Stanley (1799–1869),
British Prime Minister

There is no cure for osteoarthritis, and at present we do not have any medications or procedures that can significantly slow joint destruction. However, exercise can help to reduce joint pain and improve function. It is one of the most important activities we can undertake to help ourselves, and this chapter describes exercises for the major osteoarthritis joint groups.

The old school of thought was that exercising arthritic joints wore them out faster. Some believed that individuals had a certain number of heart beats and a certain number of steps over a lifetime and the more active one was, the sooner the joints would wear out. These theories have been disproven. In fact, low-impact activities such as walking and cycling do not accelerate articular cartilage breakdown. They are beneficial for joints, even somewhat arthritic ones. Articular cartilage needs use, and weight-bearing to knee joints pushes fluid out of the cartilage. When the weight is removed, fluids with new nutrients for articular cartilage are absorbed.

Years ago, when a patient was given a diagnosis of osteoarthritis of the knee, they were also given a prescription to be a couch potato. However, this created a group of middle-aged individuals who became sedentary, depressed, and sometimes overweight, with resulting high blood pressure and cholesterol levels. Today, for every diagnosis we make, some type of exercise program for each patient is prescribed.

WHAT ARE THE GOALS OF AN EXERCISE PROGRAM?

Exercise programs for those with osteoarthritis should be individualized. A few general exercise goals should be kept in mind: improving the strength and range of motion of the affected joints, protecting them from further damage through joint protection, and improving overall health.

Almost all exercise programs should include some type of low-impact activity to build up muscle strength without adding additional stress to the osteoarthritic joint. Examples of this include swimming or brisk walking. Individualized exercise programs might focus attention on increasing range of motion and function of small joints such as the hands, for example, or strengthening of the quadriceps muscle for knee osteoarthritis. A combination of an exercise program and physical therapy program focusing on individual joints and muscles will allow patients with osteoarthritis to experience relief from pain. Patients can increase endurance during activities, and thereby possibly delay the need for a joint replacement.

The severity of osteoarthritis at the time a patient begins an exercise program may limit positive outcomes. If a patient has severe knee osteoarthritis with complete loss of articular cartilage, there is unfortunately little that can be done for that knee joint. However, the patient can work on exercises to improve his/her overall physical fitness level. It is important that every patient's exercise program be individualized according to his/her disease severity.

Some exercises are *isotonic*, to tighten muscles by moving joints. If a patient is inflamed or finds it difficult to move joints, however, the doctor may prescribe *isometric* exercises, which tighten muscles without moving a joint. Both isometric and isotonic exercises are *aerobic* and increase oxygen consumption by the body.

EXERCISES FOR THE NECK

Neck osteoarthritis develops when discs between the neck vertebrae degenerate and small joints next to the vertebrae, the apophyseal joints or facet joints, overwork and wear out. Pain that develops with neck osteoarthritis can result from bone spurs, which grow into the canal where nerves leave the neck. This causes sharp pain to the neck and down the shoulder and arm. The facet joints can be painful and this is noticeable when moving the neck from side to side or rotating it. Muscle spasm may also be experienced next to the vertebrae in the neck, which causes pain from muscle tightness. Exercises for neck osteoarthritis are directed towards relieving the pain cycle by strengthening muscles around painful joints and increasing the range of motion of the neck.

Neck range of motion and isometric exercises

These should be done slowly at first and try to workup to a new level each day. Repeat these exercises a few times a day and over a few weeks, and try to slowly increase the range of motion. When performing resistive exercises, try to maintain the position for at least 5 seconds.

1. Look down, and bend your chin as far forward as you can to touch your chest. Next, place a hand on your forehead and try to look down and resist the head movement. You may initially experience some pain and stiffness; if this occurs, stop bending forward. (Figure 29)
2. Stand straight and look up, and try to bend your head back to look at the ceiling but do not force the movement and stop if you feel pain. Place your hand on the back of your head and try to move your head to look up, and resist this head movement. (Figure 30)
3. Tilt your head towards your left ear to your left shoulder until you feel stiffness or pain, then repeat this movement for the right ear to the right shoulder. Place your hand above your left ear and try to resist the head movement as you tilt it toward the left ear. Repeat this for the right ear. (Figure 31)
4. Turn your head to look over the left shoulder, and then turn your head to look over your right shoulder. Next, put your left hand above your left ear and resist moving your head to look over your left shoulder. (Figure 32)

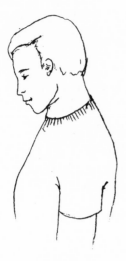

FIG. 29
Neck exercise: chin to chest

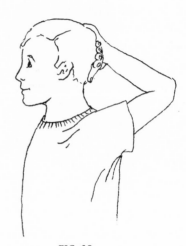

FIG. 30
Neck exercise: ceiling glance

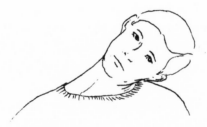

FIG. 31
Neck exercise: side tilt

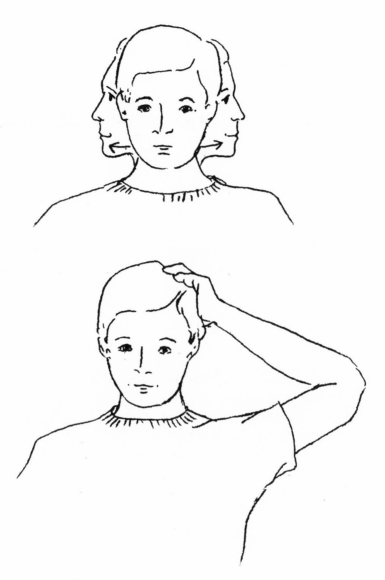

FIG. 32 *Neck exercises: side tilt (above) and head twist (below)*

EXERCISES FOR THE SHOULDER

The shoulder is held in position by a number of ligaments called the rotator cuff. When the shoulder becomes arthritic and the joint pain reduces the range of motion, the tendons and ligaments of the rotator cuff become weak. Exercises for the shoulder joint involve increasing the joint's range of motion and strengthening muscles and tendons in the rotator cuff.

Shoulder range of motion and strengthening exercises

These exercises can be performed in a standing or sitting position, depending on your comfort level.

1. Put your hands together behind your neck, then bring your elbows together in front of you, and then separate them as far apart as you can. Try to repeat this about 10 times, two to three times a day. (Figure 33)
2. Put one hand behind your back. Then put the other hand behind your back and cross the wrists, and try to stretch your hand to touch the top of your pelvic bone. Repeat this a number of times, trying to stretch your hands further each time. (Figure 34)
3. Hold both arms down at your sides, then raise the left arm straight up and reach over your head towards the ceiling. Repeat for the right arm. (Figure 35)
4. Turn your body so that your left side faces the wall. Take your left arm and slowly walk up the wall with the fingers of your left hand as far up the wall as you can go. Repeat this for the right side. Each day try to go a little further up the wall. (Figure 36)
5. Put your left arm out to side as far as it can go. Move the left arm as far up as possible without pain. Move the left hand in a circle for about three rotations. Repeat with the right arm. (Figure 37)
6. Strengthening the shoulders' girdle muscles can improve range of motion and strength in the upper arm and shoulder area. For this exercise, either use a can of soup or purchase a light free weight of one to three pounds. (Do not use more than five pounds.) Lift the weights from the side and raise them up over the head. Bend your knees slightly to avoid straining the lumbar spine. If you are unable to lift your arms above the head, you can bring your hands together on the chest and then extend the arms fully. Keep one hand on the chair to maintain your balance, and bend one knee. (Figure 38)

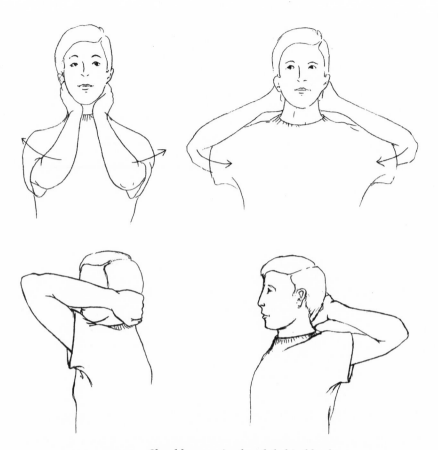

FIG. 33   *Shoulder exercise: hands behind back*

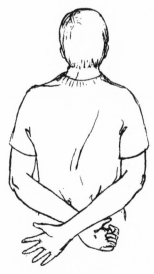

FIG. 34
Shoulder exercise: stretching to the side

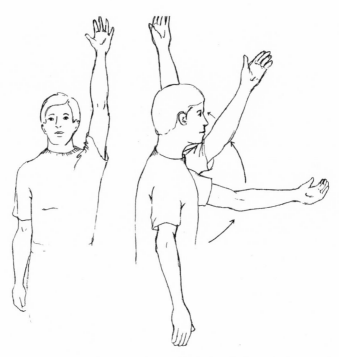

FIG. 35   *Shoulder exercise: lifting arm straight*

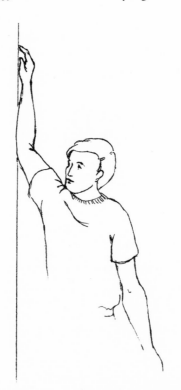

FIG. 36   *Shoulder exercise: fingers walking up a wall*

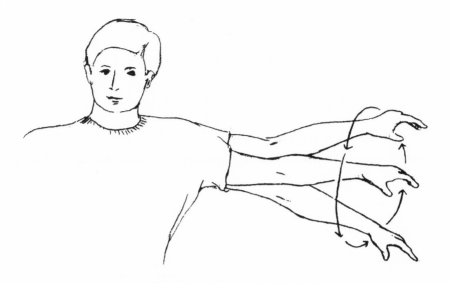

FIG. 37   *Shoulder exercise: moving hand in a circle*

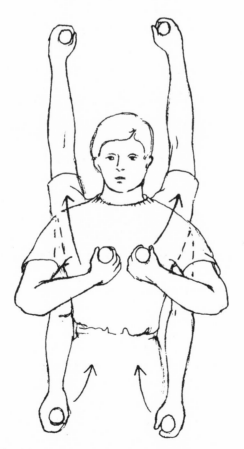

FIG. 38   *Shoulder exercise: strengthening shoulder extensor muscles*

EXERCISES FOR THE HIP

As the hip develops osteoarthritis, walking becomes becomes painful and the joint becomes stiff. It becomes difficult to bend the hip or straighten it out completely. Exercises for the hip are aimed at increasing range of motion of the joint. All the range of motion exercises are done lying on your back.

Hip range of motion exercises

1. Move your knee up and to 90 degrees and try to bend it toward your chest. Move each knee separately, and then try to move both knees at the same time. (Figure 39)
2. Bend one knee by bringing your foot in toward your buttock. Try to rotate your other leg out toward the side. Then bend the other knee. Repeat this. (Figure 40)
3. Lying on the floor on your stomach, arms next to the head, raise your left thigh straight up off the floor as far as it can go. Try to hold this position for five seconds, then switch sides. (Figure 41).

EXERCISES FOR THE KNEE

When the knee develops osteoarthritis, usually joint pain results in reduced or limited physical activity. This results in loss of strength in the quadriceps muscle in the affected leg. Exercises for knee osteoarthritis are aimed at increasing flexibility and strengthening.

Knee flexibility and strengthening exercises

1. Sit on the floor and straighten your leg as much as far as you can tolerate it. Point your toes toward your chest and tighten the muscles around your kneecap and thigh. Repeat this a few times a day. (Figure 42)
2. To strengthen quadriceps, lie on the floor and raise one leg up as far as your can, while pushing your back against the floor. When your back begins to arch, hold that position for about five seconds. Repeat this movement with the other leg. (Figure 43)

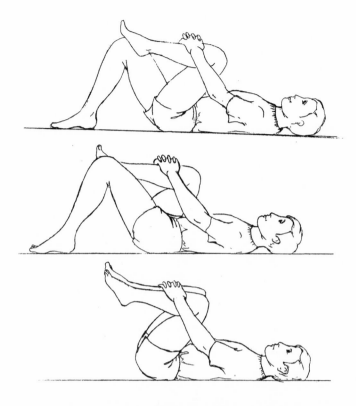

FIG. 39   *Hip exercise: knee to chest*

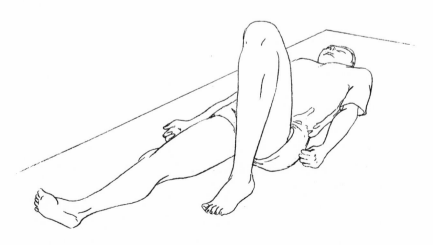

FIG. 40   *Hip exercise: knee flexing*

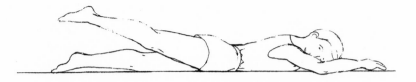

FIG. 41   *Hip exercise: leg raises*

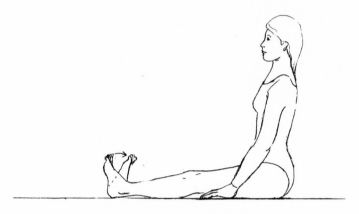

FIG. 42   *Knee exercise: leg straightening*

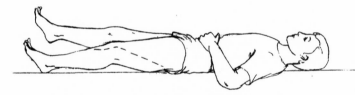

FIG. 43   *Knee exercise: quadriceps strengthening*

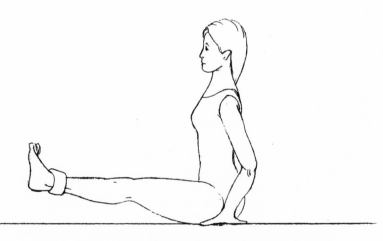

FIG. 44   *Knee exercise: leg muscle strengthening with weights*

3. Sit on the floor and support your body with your arms at your side. Put your legs out straight. Put a three-pound weight around the ankle and lift your leg a few inches off the floor and hold the position for a few seconds. Continue lowering and raising the leg with the ankle weight, while keeping the knee straight. Repeat with the other leg. Perform five or six repetitions for each leg every day. The weight on the ankle can be slowly increased over a few weeks, but should never be greater than five pounds without consulting a physician or a physical therapist. (Figure 44)

EXERCISES FOR THE SPINE

Spine or back osteoarthritis develops when discs in between the spinal vertebrae degenerate and the small joints next to the vertebrae (apophyseal and facet joints) overwork and wear out. Spinal pain results from bone spurs that grow into the canal where the nerve leaves the neck. This may produce sharp discomfort in the back and down the back of the lower leg. Facet joints can also become painful when you move or twist your lower back, bend to the side, or rotate. The pain travels from the lower back into the groin area. You may also notice some painful muscle spasms next to the lower spine vertebrae. Exercises for spine or back osteoarthritis are directed towards increasing the range of motion and strengthening back muscles.

Range of motion and strengthening exercises for the spine
Many of these exercises can also be performed by women with osteoporosis and compression vertebral fractures, because strengthening the back muscles can reduce pain and improve mobility in those situations as well.

1. Back extension exercises can be done in a sitting position. Sitting avoids or decreases pain in some patients with severe pain. These exercises should be done for five to ten minutes three times a week, and increased as tolerated. (Figure 45)
2. This back extension exercise can be done while lying on the abdomen. Lift the head and chest for a few seconds at a time. A

floor pad and pillow should be used for support. Perform this exercise for five to ten minutes three times a week, and increase as tolerated. (Figure 46)

3. This isometric exercise decreases lumbar lordosis by pulling up the abdomen. Lie on a floor mat, and with the knees bent 90 degrees, press the small of your lower back into the mat. Initially this exercise should be done slowly, five to ten repetitions in one sitting once or twice a week, and increasing to once a day. (Figure 47)

4. Lie on your back and lift the knees about 45 degrees. Then lift the head towards the chest. This exercise strengthens the abdominal muscles so that they better support an arthritic back. Initially this exercise should be done slowly, five to ten times in one sitting once or twice a week, and then increasing to once a day. (Figure 48)

5. Another exercise to strengthen the abdominal muscles is done by lying on the back and placing your hands in the space between the spine and the mat. Then lift the legs, one at a time, about 20 to 40 degrees above the pad for a few seconds and then lower them to the mat. Do this exercise slowly at first, five to ten times in one sitting once or twice a week, then increase to once a day. (Figure 49)

6. Exercises with an elastic band increase resistance and muscle strength. These exercises can strengthen the shoulder, mid-back, lower back, and hip musculature. Strengthening these muscles helps to support an arthritic spine. (Figure 50)

Place an elastic band about 2 feet long over a bar about 2 feet above your head. When you grasp either end of the band and pull down, the latissimus dorsi and shoulder adductors (upper back muscles) are strengthened. The elastic band can also be used by holding either end with one hand and standing with both feet on the middle of the band. When you pull the band backward, the shoulder adductors and extensors get a workout. When you pull your arms up over your head, the back extensor muscles are strengthened.

WHAT ABOUT EXERCISE FOR PHYSICAL FITNESS?

Exercise is important for everyone; it increases the heart rate and improves overall physical conditioning. A number of studies have found

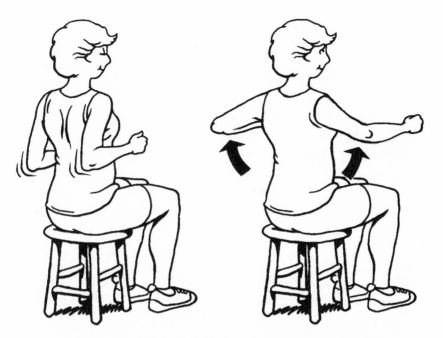

FIG. 45   *A back extension exercise*

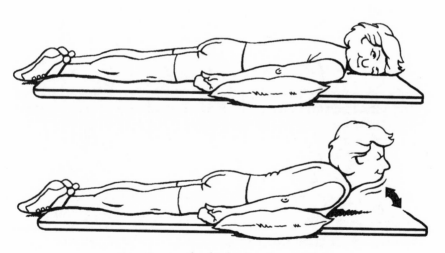

FIG. 46   *Another back extension exercise*

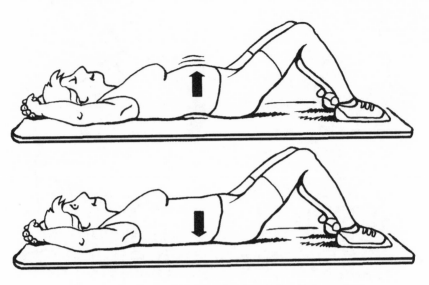

FIG. 47   *Back exercise: strengthening abdominal muscles*

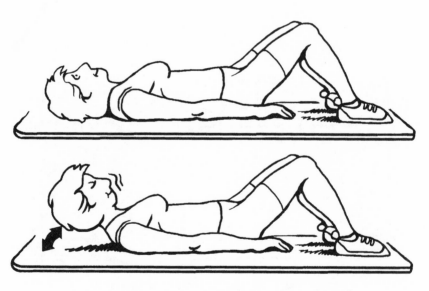

FIG. 48   *another exercise to strengthen abdominal muscles*

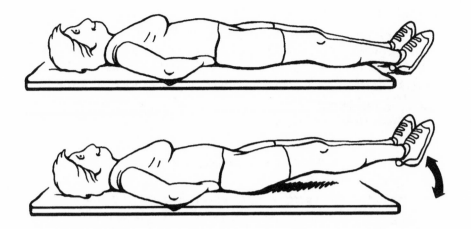

FIG. 49   *Back exercise: another exercise to strengthen abdominal muscles*

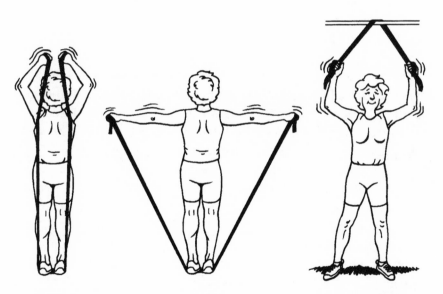

FIG. 50   *Back exercise: strengthening muscles to support an arthritic spine*

that elderly individuals regularly participating in some type of aerobic exercise program have a better quality of life and live longer than individuals who do not regularly exercise. The type of aerobic exercise that individuals undertake depends on their physical ailments. People with knee osteoarthritis usually do not like to jog, because their knees become painful. Therefore, other types of aerobic exercise are required. Some suggestions are listed below.

- *Swimming or water aerobic classes.* Places little stress on the knees and hips.
- *Walking.* A good exercise as it gives cartilage of the weight-bearing joints a chance to be exercised with very little impact and helps keep cartilage healthy.
- *Rowing or bicycling.* Places little stress on the knees and hips.
- *Exercising with a partner or a group.* Keeps interest level higher, exercises can be varied.
- *Low-impact aerobic exercise classes.* Excellent for cardiovascular fitness and low impact to weight-bearing arthritic joints.

There is no doubt that regular aerobic exercise can help improve one's mental well-being and overall physical functioning. In a study of elderly individuals with knee osteoarthritis, some were prescribed low-impact exercise a few times a week for one hour for 18 months, and some performed no exercise. The exercising patients improved physical functioning and were able to walk increased distances, while the group that just took a health education course had not improved. It is clear that a diagnosis of knee osteoarthritis or any type of osteoarthritis means that each patient should have a prescription for some type of exercise program that works with their lifestyle. These exercise programs not only improve physical functioning and quality of life, but extend the lifespan. Check with your physician or health care provider before you undertake a new exercise program to be sure that it is appropriate for your osteoarthritis and other medical conditions. It is sometimes helpful to have your doctor write a prescription for a physical therapy assessment to establish a sensible exercise course.

WHAT HAPPENS IF MY JOINTS HURT AFTER EXERCISE?

In general, you should not exercise a joint to the point of increased pain. When osteoarthritis patients initially begin an exercise program, however, joints often hurt after exercise. It is appropriate to apply an ice pack to the painful joint for about 20 minutes after exercising. You can repeat the icing several times a day if required. If you find that icing before a work-out helps to reduce pain *after* a work-out, then do this. Remember that pain is nature's way of telling us not to do something. If joint pain becomes severe after activity, it is best not to do that type of activity.

SUMMARY

We're seen that carefully tailored exercise regimens are useful for osteoarthritis sufferers. Exercise costs nothing, strengthens muscles, and if done correctly, can help prevent cartilage and joint degeneration. Consult a physician regarding the best program for you.

17

How Osteoarthritis Medications Are Tested

There are no really "safe" biologically active drugs. There are only "safe" physicians.

—Harold Kaminetzky (born 1921–)

Unlike over-the-counter drugs alternative remedies, medications approved by the Food and Drug Administration (FDA) for osteoarthritis have undergone rigorous testing in order to obtain this specific indication. Because a significant amount of irreversible joint destruction has already occurred before joint pain develops and medical attention is sought, the medications used to treat osteoarthritis today are directed towards reducing joint pain and improving joint function. Hopefully, future medications will slow or reverse the disease.

Medications developed to reduce pain and inflammation and improve function are tested in very specific ways. The FDA has guidelines that pharmaceutical companies must follow during the clinical development of osteoarthritis medications. This chapter reviews the process that candidate drugs undergo in order to receive FDA approval.

THE PRECLINICAL PROCESS: BEFORE HUMANS

The first part of medication development begins at the preclinical stage. Chemical compounds that may have anti-inflammatory or analgesic properties are evaluated in a laboratory environment to assess whether they have these effects. It is not possible to stop testing at this point, however, and thus promising compounds are further studied using living models. Laboratory animals are exposed to a painful stimulus or given a disease similar to knee osteoarthritis by cutting their anterior cruciate ligament or cutting out a piece of the meniscus, and allowing the animal to develop osteoarthritis of the knee. The animals are then given a test medication or placebo. The animals are ultimately sacrificed and the cartilage of the osteoarthritic joint is evaluated. Many nonsteroidal (aspirin and ibuprofen-like) drugs have been tested in this way. Recently, medications that may have the ability to re-grow cartilage are also being tested on animals.

Test animals are treated as humanely as possible according to set guidelines. Since thousands of chemical compounds are evaluated for every drug that makes it to the market, and some animals (such as mice) live only two years in their natural state, animal testing saves thousands of human years in developing new drugs. Thousands of life-saving medications currently on the market could never have been evaluated without using animals, as there are no other alternatives at this time.

The FDA mandates long-term safety studies in animals. During the development process, pharmaceutical companies are required to ascertain that a new medication does not cause toxic side effects to any organs of the body. Some of these safety studies can take up to two years.

An important aspect of the preclinical drug development process is that the pharmaceutical company and the FDA must determine if the medication is helpful or efficacious for human beings as well as safe in animals. In addition, the pharmaceutical company usually gets some idea of the human dose that will be needed to obtain reduction in pain and inflammation.

These preclinical studies are critical to understanding which chemical compounds are potentially useful, and, much more importantly, if they are safe enough to test in humans. The reader can log onto the FDA website for information on the osteoarthritis drug development process (see www.fda.gov).

PHASE I AND II STUDIES: EARLY OSTEOARTHRITIS DRUG TESTING IN HUMANS

Once a new medication is going to be tested in humans, there are four phases of drug development. Phase I is required by the FDA to determine if a medication is safe. This is the first time the medication will be given to small numbers of human study subjects. A Phase I trial is usually very brief, often only one to two weeks in duration. The *pharmacokinetics* of the drug (how it is absorbed, metabolized, and excreted) is looked at in detail. A major goal of a Phase I trial is to determine if the drug is safe and does not harm any organ system. These studies suggest the optimal dose of medication to use in future studies.

Phase II studies are then conducted to determine if the new osteoarthritis medication works. Which dose is most effective? Is the drug safe when given for a longer time period? In these studies blood and urine tests are obtained, as well as X-rays. A Phase II study for an osteoarthritis medication being evaluated to reduce pain and joint inflammation usually lasts around 12 to 24 weeks. During that time, patients may come to the physician's office or study clinic as often as every two weeks to provide information on their joint pain, and have blood and urine checked for safety.

PHASE III TRIALS: THE LINCHPIN AS TO WHETHER OR NOT A DRUG GETS APPROVED

Phase III studies usually involve large study groups and use the dose or doses of medications found in Phase II to work best. These studies may last anywhere from twelve weeks to as long as a year. During that time patients will come to the study center a number of times to be examined, give blood and urine samples, and fill out questionnaires about their joint pain and function. The American College of Rheumatology (ACR) has developed definitions of osteoarthritis of the hips, knees, and hands (see Table 13, at the end of the chapter). These are used as minimal inclusion criteria for participation in Phase II, III, and IV clinical trials. The study subject will usually have an X-ray of the affected joint and a blood test to make sure they are healthy enough for the study. Once they qualify, they will usually be asked to stop their current osteoarthritis medication. When their knee pain, for example, increases to a certain level or they experience a "flare-up" the patient will be asked to come to the study center. At this point the patient will receive either the study medication or an inactive placebo. In a typical Phase III study, the subject will return every few weeks for a few visits, after which the visits will take place at longer intervals. A Phase III study is meant to be wide-ranging and is usually conducted in many centers and often in different countries. When all of the study subjects have completed the clinical trial and all the data and laboratory findings have been returned to the pharmaceutical company and analyzed, the information is given to the FDA for approval. There are many different things that the FDA looks for when reviewing study results. Their most important concern is, of course, the medication's safety. The FDA will also look at each study to determine if the new medication was effective. Did it decrease joint pain or inflammation, and improve the quality of life of the patient with osteoarthritis? In addition, the FDA will look to see if certain groups of patients with osteoarthritis improved more than others. For new osteoarthritis medications, the requirements are that the medication is safe, and that it reduces pain and inflammation in the osteoarthritic joint more than an inactive medication or placebo.

After the FDA reviews the study results, an advisory panel is formed for further review. These panel experts do not work for the FDA. If the advisory panel approves the medication, then the next step is to write a label for the new medication. The pharmaceutical company works with the FDA to provide a detailed package label. The label describes the chemicals in the medication, all of the studies that were performed, what the drug is approved for, and potential side effects the drug can cause. It also explains how to dose the medication, and any precautions that need to be taken if a patient is also taking other medication. It is not unusual for the agreement and writing of the the package label to take months to accomplish.

PHASE IV STUDIES: ICING ON THE CAKE AFTER A DRUG IS APPROVED

After a drug receives FDA approval, Phase IV studies can be conducted. These are often competitive in nature in that they compare one drug to another competing drug. (Phase IV trials do not usually involve an inactive medication or placebo.) In a study for osteoarthritis medications, an example would be to test ibuprofen (Motrin or Advil) against naproxen (Naprosyn, Aleve) or celecoxib (Celebrex). The goal of a competitive study is to ascertain if two or three drugs are equivalent or if one is superior. Another type of Phase IV study is to obtain a new approved category of use for an already approved medication. For example, if a medication was approved for the signs and symptoms of osteoarthritis, additional

Table 12: How the osteoarthritis prescription drug evaluation process works

Preclinical Stage

Compounds are tested in the laboratory for anti-inflammatory properties or suggestions of analgesic properties, and those that are promising are tested in animals.

Phase I Testing

Drugs are tested in a small number of humans for a short period of time in a variety of doses as part of a pharmacokinetic and safety evaluation, to ascertain how the drug is tolerated and handled by the liver, kidney, and gastrointestinal tract.

Phase II Testing

Agents are tested in 5–20 centers in around 50 people, for 3–6 months, in a few dosing regimens.

Phase III Testing

Agents are tested in a wide-ranging study of patients and in different locations for up to a year.

Phase IV Testing

After FDA approval, a Phase IV trial (a.) provides long-term follow up on Phase III patients; (b.) evaluates the drug for a different disease or use; or (c.) compares it to other agents approved for the same use.

studies would be performed to receive an approval for the signs and symptoms of rheumatoid arthritis. Or, a drug approved to reduce pain in osteoarthritis might be determined to be useful for premenstrual pain. Sometimes, those studying Phase IV work with the same patients enrolled during Phase III, to obtain information concerning long-term safety or efficacy.

SUMMARY: HOW MUCH SHOULD AN OSTEOARTHRITIS DRUG COST?

Getting a new medication approved for osteoarthritis has many steps (summarized in Table 12). The development process starts before the medication is used in humans. Then there are four phases in which the medication is tested, and it cannot be approved for use by the public until the first three phases are performed. The job of the FDA is to make sure that pharmaceutical companies follow the correct process, interpret all the study results correctly, keep safety in mind, and provide the public with new, more effective medications as expeditiously as possible. The process of reviewing a new medication can be complex, and new arthritis drugs may take two to ten years and cost the manufacturer between 80 and 300 million dollars to develop. Thousands of compounds tested in the laboratory result in only one or two making it to clinical trials. A minority of drugs tested in Phase I ever get approved. Drug companies have patent protection, meaning that they cannot have generic competition for 17 years from the time they file to study a new drug. Federal regulations and research costs, plus the high failure rate of drugs being studied, result in us paying what seems to be a lot of money for our medicine.

Table 13: The American College of Rheumatology criteria for osteoarthritis. These must be fulfilled in order for a patient to participate in an osteoarthritis drug study.

Hand osteoarthritis
Hand pain, aching and stiffness, and 3 of the following features:
> hard tissue enlargement of 2 or more of 10 selected joints
> hard tissue enlargement of 2 or more DIP joints
> fewer than 3 swollen MCP joints
> deformity of 1 of 10 selected joints

Hip osteoarthritis
Hip pain, and 2 of the following features:
> normal sedimentation rate
> femoral or acetabular osteophytes on X-ray
> joint space narrowing on X-ray

Knee osteoarthritis
Knee pain, and 5 of the following:
> age over 50
> stiffness lasting less than 30 minutes,
> crepitus
> bony tenderness
> bony enlargment
> no palpable warmth
> sedimentation rate less than 40
> Class I synovial fluid
> negative rheumatoid factor

OR, 1 of the following
  age over 50
  stiffness lasting less than 30 minutes
  crepitus *and* osteophytes
OR 3 of the following:
  age over 50
  stiffness lasting less than 30 minutes
  crepitus
  bony tenderness
  bony enlargment
  no palpable warmth

Sources: Altman, R Alarcon, G, and Appelrouth D et al., *The American College of Rheumatology criteria for the classification and reporting of osteoarthritis of the hand* (1990) 33: 1601–1610, and (1991) 34:505–514; Altman, Asch, and Bloch, et al., *Development of criteria for the classification and reporting of osteoarthritis: classification of osteoarthritis of the knee,* (1986) 29: 1039–1049.

18

Medications that Work for Osteoarthritis

The desire to take medicine is perhaps the greatest feature which distinguishes man from animals.
—Sir William Osler (1849–1919),
Teaching and Thinking,
Montreal Medical Journal 23:561, (1894–5)

Thus far, we have reviewed treatments of osteoarthritis that do not involve taking medicine. While diet, exercise, assistive devices, and behavioral modification play an important role, the fact remains that medication is perhaps the most important intervention we have available. By the time an osteoarthritis patient needs to take a medicine for their discomfort, articular cartilage damage can be extensive. There are no medications available to rebuild articular cartilage or slow its degeneration. Osteoarthritis does not shorten an individual's lifespan, but it can make it less enjoyable. This chapter will review the two major classes of drugs used to manage osteoarthritis: acetaminophen and the nonsteroidal anti-inflammatory drugs (NSAIDS). Subsequent chapters will discuss local and topical treatments, pain killers, alternative treatments, and surgery.

ACETAMINOPHEN

In 1995, the American College of Rheumatology recommended that acetaminophen should be considered the first drug of choice in managing mild to moderate osteoarthritis. The drug has come a long way from its humble beginnings in 1886, when a derivative of the chemical acetanilid was marketed as "antifebrin," based on its ability to decrease fevers. A variety of relatively toxic preparations were available for years as phenacetins and para-aminophenol. In 1949, an active metabolite of anetanalid and phenacitin was marketed as acetaminophen (also known as paracetamol and by the brand name Tylenol).

Acetaminophen has well-documented analgesic (pain killing) and antipyretic (fever lowering) properties. It has little anti-inflammatory action. Some osteoarthritis patients have a lot of inflammation and others have very little. In one study, acetaminophen was found to be just as effective as ibuprofen in reducing knee osteoarthritis joint pain after a month of treatment, and had fewer side effects. The drug is extremely well tolerated. Occasionally, when patients take up to four grams of acetaminophen a day, liver problems can occur and a physician will monitor this with monthly blood tests. Patients with pre-existing liver disease should be very careful about using acetaminophen. The standard prescription is two tablets at a time (or one extra strength pill) up to four times a day. Many individuals with mild osteoarthritis require only an occasional acetaminophen. Because of its relative nontoxicity acetaminophen should be the first drug a new osteoarthritis patient tries.

As good as acetaminophen can be for mild to moderate osteoarthritis, it does have limitations. As osteoarthritis worsens, simple analgesics are no longer sufficient to control joint pain, and additional interventions are needed. In one study of patients with moderate osteoarthritis, only 14% of those started on acetaminophen alone were still taking it as their only intervention after a year.

ASPIRIN AND NSAIDS: THEY WORK, BUT BE CAREFUL!

Derived from willow bark, aspirin became commercially available in 1899. Attempts to broaden its range of actions led to the synthesis of the first nonsteroidal anti-inflammatory drug (NSAID), phenylbutazone, which was approved for use in the United States in 1951. This was followed by indomethacin (1965) and ibuprofen (1974). Over 20 aspirin and NSAID derivatives were available in the United States by late 1998.

By inhibiting a chemical known as prostaglandin E2, via the enzyme cyclooxygenase (COX), aspirin and NSAIDs have four principal mechanisms of action: analgesic, antipyretic, anti-inflammatory, and blood thinning. It is clear that these drugs were just as effective as acetaminophen in managing mild osteoarthritis. In patients with inflammation and more advanced disease, they are more effective. Further, they can be used with acetaminophen. Certain patterns have evolved with aspirin and NSAIDS over the years. Many patients take occasional NSAIDs as over-the-counter preparations such as Advil or Aleve, have few problems, and therefore never see a doctor about their arthritis. However, when patients take higher doses of NSAIDs or needed them on a daily basis, problems begin to appear. NSAIDs are associated with numerous side effects. The most common are gastrointestinal in the form of heartburn, stomach ache, or nausea. Most of the time these complaints are not associated with any pathology. One regular-dosage NSAID user in 30 (3%) is admitted to the hospital each year for a gastrointestinal bleed, and high-dose regular use of NSAIDs have also been shown to affect liver and kidney function in 1-3% of individuals. By the mid-1990s, a large-scale survey estimated that the use of NSAIDs were responsible for 100,000 excess hospitalizations and 10,000 excess deaths in the United States each year. This, in part, explains why in 1995 the American College of Rheumatology advised that NSAIDs only be used for more serious cases of osteoarthritis, or when a less irritating choice such as Tylenol simply does not work. See Table 14 (at the end of the chapter) for a list of these drugs.

NONACETYLATED SALICYLATES AND PROTON PUMP INHIBITORS

In an attempt to improve the safety of aspirin and NSAIDs, several breakthroughs have been achieved to decrease their attendant risks. Doctors advise individuals taking these drugs not to smoke or drink, not to lie down after a big meal, and minimize the use of caffeine; doses are also decreased in patients over the age of 65. Patients taking corticosteroids or anticoagulants are at especially higher risks for gastrointestinal complications.

A group of aspirin-like derivatives, known as nonacetylated salicylates, were introduced in the 1960s. Under the names Disalcid, Trilisate, Magan, and Salsalate, these agents are able to decrease the gastrointestinal risks of aspirin by over 90%. Unfortunately, they are also relatively weak and can cause ringing in the ears in many patients. Nevertheless, they are at least as effective as acetaminophen. Although over-the-counter heartburn preparations such as Zantac, Axid, or Pepcid (known in medical terminology as H2-blockers) are able to greatly decrease gastrointestinal symptoms induced by NSAIDs, they do not decrease the incidence of ulcers, perforations, or bleeds. They sometimes, in fact, mask stomach symptoms, leading to more bleeding. In the late 1980s, two new types of drugs were introduced that were an improvement. The prostaglandin derivative misoprostol (under the brand name Cytotec) and proton pump inhibitors (such as Prilosec, Prevacid, Protonix, Nexium, and Aciphex) can be taken with aspirin or NSAIDs, and largely prevent the development of gastrointestinal complications. This does increase the cost of taking NSAIDs, however, and these drugs do have some minor side effects of their own.

SELECTIVE COX-2 BLOCKERS: A PROMISING ALTERNATIVE

Aspirin and NSAIDs block an enzyme known as COX, which is responsible for tissue inflammation. In the early 1990s, scientists discovered that there were two kinds of this enzyme. While aspirin and the NSAIDs available at the time nonselectively blocked both COX-1 and COX-2, it was discovered that certain new preparations could block COX-2 with little inhibition of COX-1. These selective COX-2 blockers were equally anti-inflammatory, analgesic, and antipyretic, but lacked the blood-thinning properties of nonselective COX blockers. Introduced in 1998 and 1999 as celecoxib (the brand name Celebrex) and rofecoxib (Vioxx), this new generation of drugs decreases gastrointestinal symptoms associated with NSAIDs by 90% and complications such as perforations, ulcerations, and bleeds by over 50%. Patients at high risk can further decrease their chance for gastrointestinal complications by taking proton pump inhibitors or misoprostol. In 2000, the American College of Rheumatology revised their guidelines to recommend that this class of drugs may be preferred to aspirin and NSAIDs in treating osteoarthritis pain and managing inflammatory manifestations of the disease. Though these drugs are still covered by patent and available only as brand names, they are still less expensive in that patients rarely also require proton pump inhibitors or misoprostol (which are more expensive). The result is many dollars saved in hospitalization costs. Prescriptions for COX-2 selective blockers are best restricted to patients who must take an arthritis drug every day

Table 14: Major nonsteroidal anti-inflammatory drugs (NSAIDS)

Salicylates
    Aspirin
    Sodium salicylate (Trilisate, Disalcid, Salsalate)
    Magnesium salicylate (Magan, Doan's)

Non-selective cyclooxygenase inhibitors
    Proprionic acid derivatives
        Oxaprozin (Daypro)
        Naproxen (Naprosyn, Anaprox, Aleve)
        Flurbiprofen (Ansaid)
        Ibuprofen (Motrin, Advil)
        Ketoprofen (Orudis, Oruvail)
        Fenoprofen (Nalfon)
    Acetic acid derivatives
        Sulindac (Clinoril)
        Diclofenac (Voltaren, Arthrotec, Cataflam)
        Tolmetin (Tolectin)
        Indomethacin (Indocin)
    Oxicam derivatives
        Piroxicam (Feldene)
        Meloxicam (Mobic) <A "preferential" cox-2 inhibitor
    Others
        Etodolac (Lodine)
        Ketrolac (Toradol)
        Nabumetone (Relafen)
        Meclofenates (Meclomen, Ponstel)

Selective cyclooxygenase (COX-2) inhibitors
        Celecoxib (Celebrex)
        Rofecoxib (Vioxx)

and are at higher risks for gastrointestinal toxicity. Patients taking concurrent corticosteroids or with a history of cardiovascular disease might wish to add a baby aspirin to their Cox-2 regimen.

WHAT ABOUT PAIN KILLERS?

There are times when analgesics other than NSAIDs, aspirin, or acetaminophen are needed to treat arthritis pain. Some are used locally, and others are systemic. These are reviewed in chapters 19 and 20.

SUMMARY

Acetaminophen alleviates osteoarthritis pain, while aspirin and NSAIDs diminish both pain and inflammation. Most doctors start with acetaminophen, evolve to occasional over-the-counter NSAIDs in low doses, with or without acetaminophen if the patient requires it, and prescribe NSAIDs for moderate to severe osteoarthritis. There is evidence that selective COX-2-inhibiting NSAIDs are also effective, and safer than nonselective inhibitors.

19

Local Medical Therapies

Is there no balm in Gilead; is there no physician there?
—Jeremiah 8:22

"Doctor, my knee really hurts. Isn't there something I can do locally without taking pills?" "Can't you just give me a cortisone shot?" "I've heard that there is something safer than cortisone that you can inject. Is that true?" We hear at least one of these questions daily from our patients. And the answer, fortunately, is yes. This chapter will review treatments that approach osteoarthritis with local medications.

TOPICAL ANTI-INFLAMMATORIES

Arthritis patients have applied salves and ointments to painful joints since antiquity. Paraffin, camphor, and menthol preparations are soothing and provide temporary pain relief. Unfortunately, they do nothing about the underlying problem. Over the years, some drug companies have marketed topical products that contained salicylate-based (aspirin) products with camphor or menthol (e.g., Ben Gay). These combinations have mild anti-inflammatory effects and are well tolerated.

Nonsteroidal anti-inflammatory drugs have been on the market since phenylbutazone was first approved in 1952. Over twenty NSAIDs have appeared since that time and have been available as pills, tablets, and liquid suspensions, as well as intravenous and intramuscular preparations.

While none were marketed for topical or local use in the United States, in some countries gels accounted for half of all NSAID sales. Sold also as creams, foams, patches, or sprays, these NSAIDS proved to be popular, well-tolerated, and effective for regional pain.

What happened in the United States? In order for a topical preparation of an existing approved medication to be approved for arthritis, it must conform to very complicated guidelines. As the absorption of a topical application is highly variable because surface areas are not constant, many NSAID companies found it impossible to meet FDA requirements. In the mid–1990s, however, many of the early NSAIDs lost their patent protection and became available as generic. As a consequence, some were reformulated by compounding pharmacists (specially licensed professionals who are permitted to use the chemical powder of a drug in an alternate form) as gels and legally produced for local use.

What do we know about NSAID gels? They work, and patients like them. The most common preparations are ketoprofen (the chemical in Orudis or Oruvail) and diclofenac (the chemical in Voltaren or Arthrotec), compounded at a strength of 10 or 20% in a gel. They are usually applied to a painful joint twice daily. For individuals with additional problems such as fibromyalgia, muscle relaxants (such as cyclobenzaprine, or Flexeril) or nerve medicines (e.g., carbazemine, or Tegretol) can be added to the compound. Studies have shown that although plasma levels of NSAID gels are 20–100 times less than achieved with tablets, synovial (joint) fluid levels are 60% of what is obtained orally. Topical gels rarely, if ever, cause any gastrointestinal discomfort.

Are there downsides with using topical NSAID gels? Of course. First, they tend to be rather expensive, and many insurance plans to do not pay for them. The quality of the preparations varies with the competence of the compounder. A small percentage of users complain of hypersensitivity reactions, and local irritation occasionally occurs. The gels may ruin clothes or stain fabrics, patients with hand deformities or arthritis may find them difficult to apply, and sometimes they can get messy.

Who should use a topical NSAID gel? Patients with osteoarthritis limited to one to two areas, who wish to avoid drug interactions or the side effects associated with NSAIDs—and those willing to undertake the expense.

CAPSAICIN (TOPICAL CAYENNE PEPPER)

Capsaicin is extracted from seeds and membranes of the nightshade family of plants, including the common pepper plant. One of the mediators of arthritis pain is substance P. When applied topically, capsaicin promotes the release of substance P and prevents its reaccumulation. In other words, through the net depletion of substance P, arthritis pain improves. Studies have confirmed that capsaicin is an effective vehicle in managing local osteoarthritis discomfort. Capsaicin has to be used carefully. First, it takes about a week to become effective. Second, it can produce topical burning at first in some users, and continuously in others. Areas around the eyes and mucous membranes should be avoided. A variety of capsaicin preparations are commercially available in several potencies without prescription (e.g., Dolorac and Zostrix). Capsaicin is particularly effective for patients with post-herpetic neuralgia (shingles pain). About 20% of the patients who try capsaicin for osteoarthritis pain find it to be helpful and use it fairly regularly.

JOINT INJECTIONS WITH STEROIDS

Shortly after cortisone became available in 1948, one of the pioneers of rheumatology, Joseph Hollander, began studying the use of steroid preparations for injection directly into joints. Over a ten-year trial and error period of experimentation, several early, short-acting compounds fell by the wayside and were replaced with longer-acting, or "depo" preparations. A handful of combinations stood the test of time and are currently used for joint injections. What do corticosteroids do in joints? Normally used with a local anasthetic such as xylocaine, intra-acrticular steroids act as anti-inflammatory agents. Crystals generated as part of osteoarthritis-related pseudo-gout are dissolved. Inflammatory arthritis is ameliorated. Some patients without inflammation also report improvement after steroid injections. This may be due in part to other factors; for instance, steroids injected into joints decrease metalloproteinase synthesis, which acts to protect cartilage. They also decrease the synthesis of hyaluronic acid and secretion of certain other synovial chemicals. Steroid injections are used locally when one or two joints account for the majority of overall discomfort. Most effective when inflammation is present, injections can provide weeks, months, or permanent relief.

Which preparation should be used? This decision is up to your doctor. As noted in Table 15, some work faster but don't last as long. The Kenalog steroid injection, for example, is avoided in patients where there is little soft tissue or padding, since it can induce skin atrophy or pitting of the skin. The steroid Aristospan is in an oil base (as opposed to a water base) and although it takes longer to work, it has the advantage of few side effects. (If you are systemically inflamed, however, Aristospan will not be helpful. It also costs twice as much as other preparations.) Complicated steroid injections are best administered by a physician with expertise in musculoskeletal diseases. Temporary flares of arthritis occur in some patients 12 to 36 hours post-injection, due to steroid crystals forming in joints. Flushing and tingling are prominent for a day or two in patients who receive Depo-Medrol. Sepsis, or a joint infection resulting from a steroid injection, is extremely rare, occurring in only one out of 20,000 injections.

Repeated steroid injections are not always advisable. It has been suggested that injecting the same joint more than four times a year accelerates cartilage degeneration. Failure to respond to steroid and drug therapies is an indication for orthopedic evaluation for consideration of arthroscopy or other surgical options.

HYALURONAN INJECTIONS

Hyaluronan is a normal constituent of joint fluid which helps the joint absorb shock. Responsible for the visco-elastic properties of joint fluid (stickiness), it has been suggested that viscosupplementation—a process in which sodium hyaluronate is injected locally into a joint— helps arthritis pain by restoring the viscosity of joint fluid. It may also decrease the deterioration of cartilage. Two preparations of intra-articular sodium hyaluronate, Synvisc and Hyalgan, are approved by the FDA for patients with osteoarthritis of the knee that are unresponsive to analgesic therapies. Injected weekly for three to five weeks, the treatment course is expensive. It costs five to ten times what intra-articular steroids do, requires more than one visit, and there is no evidence they are more effective. In fact, naproxen (Naprosyn or Aleve) is as efficacious as hyaluronate injections in relieving knee pain.

When do we recommend viscosupplementation? Synvisc and Hyalgan are used to buy time for patients who need a knee replacement. It is

Table 15: Local medical therapies

Topical applications for osteoarthritis
    Containing anti-inflammatories (salicylates, NSAIDS)
    Containing soothing substances (camphor, menthol)
    Capsaisin

Nonsteroid joint injections for osteoarthritis
    Hyaluronan injections (Synvisc, Hyalgan)
    Radiosynovectomy (injection of radioactive substances, used in Europe)

Steroid injections into the joint
    Hydrocortisone (weak, short acting)
    Depo-Medrol, methylprednisolone (high systemic levels of steroids,
    works for 1–2 weeks)
    Kenalog, Aristocort, triamcinolone (moderate systemic levels of steroids,
    works for 4–16 weeks)
    Celestone, betamethasone (moderate systemic levels of steroids, works
    for 2–8 weeks, safest in pregnancy)
    Aristospan, triamcinolone (little systemic levels of steroids, takes a week
    to be effective and lasts for months, oil base, expensive)
    Decadron LA, dexamethasone (moderate systemic levels of steroids,
    works for 2–6 weeks)

also used in individuals who tolerate local steroids poorly (e.g., diabetics) or receive few benefits from oral analgesic or anti-inflammatory medications. The injection series can give some patients up to a year of relief, at which point the process can be repeated. About 20% of those who receive hyaluronate have a demonstrable, long-term, favorable response. The injections are generally well tolerated. Up to 15% of the time a mild, post-injection flare may occur which lasts a day or two. Most patients start to respond within one or two weeks.

OTHER LOCAL THERAPIES

Radiosynovectomy (irradiating an inflamed joint) is a procedure used in Europe, but has been disappointing in osteoarthritis. Laser therapy to degenerated joints has not yet been well studied. Taping, joint lavage, and arthroscopy are reviewed in chapters 15 and 21, and alternative therapies in chapter 22.

SUMMARY

Various local medical therapies are available to ameliorate osteoarthritis. Topical anti-inflammatory gels (NASAIDS) and capsaicin (derived from the pepper plant) have proved effective for some patients, while joint injections with steroids can provide relief for others.

20

But Doctor, I'm in Pain!

Culture makes pain tolerable by interpreting its necessity, only pain perceived as curable is intolerable.
—Ivan Illich, *Medical Nemesis* (1976)

Pain is the most common symptom which brings osteoarthritis to a patient's (and doctor's) attention. It is far more frequently noted than fatigue, stiffness, or muscle weakness. There are many causes of osteoarthritis pain, and its management depends on the source. This chapter will review the reasons why osteoarthritis patients experience pain and what can be done about it.

WHY DO I HURT?

The International Association for the Study of Pain has defined pain as an unpleasant sensory and cultural experience. Some patients with osteoarthritis have no symptoms, yet others complain of mild to severe pain. Why is this the case? Pain is usually experienced with joint loading and relieved with rest. A variety of factors contribute to the perception of pain in osteoarthritis (shown in Figure 51). The synovial membrane or joint lining might not get enough oxygen, limiting the blood flow. This causes bone angina. Subchondral pressure microfractures also can produce discomfort. Osteophytes cause painful sensations when they press on sensory nerves, or when the periosteum is elevated. Inflamed

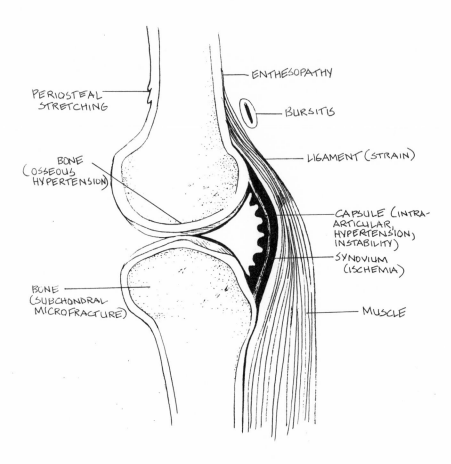

PERIOSTEAL
STRETCHING

ENTHESOPATHY

BURSITIS

LIGAMENT (STRAIN)

BONE
(OSSEOUS
HYPERTENSION)

CAPSULE (INTRA-
ARTICULAR,
HYPERTENSION,
INSTABILITY)

SYNOVIUM
(ISCHEMIA)

BONE
(SUBCHONDRAL
MICROFRACTURE)

MUSCLE

FIG. 51   *Causes of joint pain in osteoarthritis*

joint capsules, tendons, or bursa can stretch, raising bone pressure or producing instability. Nerves that traverse joints can be compressed or compromised, producing a neurogenic discomfort. Calcium deposits in joints or bursae may crystallize. Muscles around affected joints may experience reactive spasms, which sometimes entrap nerves. The indirect release of enzymes and other inflammatory mediators from cartilage stimulates a low-grade inflammatory reaction. Joint instability, locking, and torn or degenerated tissues such as menisci or ligaments can all produce pain. And the destruction of cartilage, which causes bone to rub against bone, also leads to excruciating discomfort.

HOW PAIN MAKES ITSELF FELT

Osteoarthritis is a disease of cartilage. Nerves transmit pain signals, but cartilage has no nerve fibers. How then does pain make itself felt? Picture our nerve fibers as an electrical circuit board. Wires connect the periphery to the spinal cord. Whereas pressure, heat, touch, and other sensations activate certain sensors or receptors under the skin, some of these and other sensors are known as *nociceptors*.

A nociceptor is a receptor that is sensitive to a noxious or unpleasant stimulus. Nociceptors are present in blood vessel walls, muscle, fascia, tendons, joint capsules, fat pads, synovial fluid, and body surfaces. Nociception is transmitted to the spinal cord by thin, uninsulated *unmyelinated Type C fibers*. A chemical known as *substance P* and another chemical called *calcitonin-related gene peptide* (CGRP) are present in increased amounts in the synovium of patients with osteoarthritis, and these augment pain sensations. Type C fibers traverse the musculoskeletal tissues to an area in the rear of the spinal cord known as the dorsal horn ganglion. In the dorsal horn, chemicals known as *neuropeptides* are released, including more substance P and CGRP. Another set of wires transmits nociceptive signals to spinal cord nerve cells, and then travel up to the brain. The brain interprets these messages and secretes a substance known as *endorphin*, which can mute or eliminate pain. It sends signals back down the spinal column via *adrenaline* and *serotonin*, the principal neurotransmitters of the descending system.

BEHAVIORAL APPROACHES TOWARD COPING WITH PAIN

Pain is subjective. It's not visible. The degree of pain one is aware of is dependent upon a variety of factors such as behavioral patterns (personality, mood, attitude) and sociological factors (work, economic status, culture, family relationships). These factors interact with neuropeptides to alter pain perception. Its management involves merging medication, psychological, and physical approaches.

From the anatomic standpoint, we react to osteoarthritis pain by reflex actions. In knee osteoarthritis, these reflexes include guarding, unloading a joint, rigidity, and joint flexing. Because osteoarthritis is associated with certain predictors of depression, however, these physical reflexes alone cannot determine how a patient will cope with pain. More pain is associated with passive coping strategies, such as catastrophisizing (thinking that nothing will improve the situation), escapist fantasies, avoidance, or social withdrawal.

The better way to deal with the pain associated with osteoarthritis is to work towards decreasing physical disabilities and educating oneself about the disease. Behavioral strategies are successful in diminishing discomfort. Attention diversion, for instance, includes relaxation techniques, visual imagery, and other activities to distract one from being aware of pain. It may also be helpful to encourage patients to try and sublimate painful sensations. Changing activity patterns—such as promoting periods of activity alternating with periods of rest—are also useful. All of these are positive, constructive approaches. It's important not to be a martyr to pain.

WHAT PAIN MEDICINE SHOULD I TAKE?

The correct treatment for osteoarthritis pain depends on its cause. Although a positive attitude toward dealing with pain and lifestyle is important, it is sometimes necessary to take medicines for pain as well. Most osteoarthritis patients don't need to take pain medicine all the time. For certain types of discomfort, occasional or intermittent use is all that is required. The several types of osteoarthritis pain and medications for management are listed in Table 16, at the end of the chapter.

Osteoarthritis pain due to inflammation

Synovitis, (inflammation of the joint) is found to a clinically significant degree in about half of all individuals with osteoarthritis. The extreme form of this takes place when calcium pyrophosphate crystallizes, as seen in pseudo-gout. Acetaminophen is worthless for inflammatory arthritis. Nonsteroidal anti-inflammatory agents and aspirin derivatives are the therapy of choice, preferably those that do not damage cartilage. We prefer the new selective cox-2 inhibitors, (such as Celebrex, and Vioxx.) When pseudo-gout supervenes, the usual recommended daily dose may be doubled for a few days. Inflammatory pain resistant to nonsteroidals frequently responds to local injections of corticosteroids with an anesthetic, such as xylocaine or marcaine.

Osteoarthritis pain due to degeneration or impairment of structural integrity

Cartilage degeneration, joint instability, torn menisci, osteophytic pressure, lack of blood flow to the synovium, and alterations in the structures of tendons or ligaments are the most common causes of pain in osteoarthritis. This type of pain responds to acetaminophen, as well as aspirin and the nonsteroidals. Numerous studies published before selective cox-2 inhibitors were approved in late 1998 suggested that Tylenol was safer and more cost-effective. Recent suggestions that selective cox-2 inhibitors are excellent analgesics, as safe as Tylenol, and more effective, will result in this issue being revisited. Splinting, bracing, assistive devices, and exercise programs diminish pain, as do pacing activities, physical therapy and occupational therapy. Corticosteroid injections can be somewhat helpful, but they do not work for everyone. Injecting the same joint more than four times a year can denude cartilage, and if this frequency becomes necessary, then surgical options should be considered. Injections into the joint of hyaluronate preparations usually provide modest relief for several months.

Occasionally, osteoarthritis pain does not adequately respond to any of these regimens. In these circumstances, your doctor may prescribe an analgesic painkiller that is safe, cost-effective, and nonaddictive. No currently available drug fits this bill entirely. Tramadol (the brand name Ultram) is a preparation that raises serotonin and noradrenalin levels and blocks several pain pathways. It is effective, safe in low doses, and nonaddictive, but more costly than time-honored alternatives which include the occasional or low dose use of aspirin or acetaminophen with codeine (e.g., Tylenol #3), propoxyphene (Darvon Compound, Darvocet), hydrocodone (Vicodin, or Vicoprofen with ibuprofen), or pentazocine (Talacen). All these agents are potentially addictive, and can cause constipation and dulling of the senses. We tend to use them in patients awaiting orthopedic surgery, at bedtime to aid restful sleep, and in post-operative settings.

Muscular pain

Occasionally, osteoarthritic changes are associated with muscular spasms and referred regional pain. A coexisting fibromyalgia may also be present, which can be aggravated by osteoarthritis (or difficult to differentiate). In these circumstances, tricyclic antidepressants, which have muscle relaxant properties, might be added at bedtime. Examples of these are cyclobenzaprine (Flexeril), doxepin (Sinequan), or amitriptyline (Elavil). In some patients, benzodiazepines such as clonazepam (Klonopin) may be preferable. For daytime use, muscular spasms can be modestly alleviated by orphenadine (Norgesic), carisoprodol (Soma), or methocarbamol (Robaxin). Many of these preparations are also available as combinations with acetaminophen or aspirin.

I CAN'T STAND THE PAIN ANY LONGER!

Painful osteoarthritis is divided into acute and chronic types. Examples of acute pain include pseudo-gout or a herniated disc resulting from osteoarthritis changes. The latter might be managed with bed rest, local steroid injections, nonsteroidal anti-inflammatory drugs, and analgesics. Epidural blocks with corticosteroids may also be helpful, and surgery is occasionally advised.

On the other hand, the management of chronic pain has become a controversial problem. If one has a bone-on-bone situation and there is essentially no cartilage remaining, surgery is usually recommended. When patients are not medically stable for surgery, or must delay it for personal reasons, we frequently use the analgesic regimens. The amount of pain may be so severe that narcotic analgesics such as morphine derivatives (MS contin, Oxycontin), meperidine (Demerol), time-release narcotic patches (Fentanyl), or oxycodone (Percodan, Percocet) may be prescribed. These agents are addictive, cause constipation, do not always work that well, may produce mental clouding, and can have a rebound effect if not formulated as a time-released preparation.

The "chronic pain" debate

George had such severe low back pain he could not sleep. An MRI showed bulging discs, but little in the way of clear-cut spine pathology. When anti-inflammatory drugs had no effect, he underwent three epidural blocks a week apart. The improvement was temporary. George's pain was so profound that when a myelogram suggested a slight spinal cord compression, Dr. Smith performed spinal surgery to relieve the pressure. It worked for three weeks. George needed to take up to eight Vicodan a day to function. Repeat imaging studies suggested that his lumbar fusion had failed, and he underwent a second surgery. He went to a pain specialist who prescribed a fentanyl (72-hour time-release morphine) patch. His pain diminshed slightly. At this point, George was sent by the pain specialist to a comprehensive rehabilitation program at the local hospital. As part of the evaluation, a rheumatology consultation was requested. Apparently, nobody had performed a thorough complete physical examination. Dr. James diagnosed George as having fibromyalgia. Though every part of the body was tender to touch, tender points in the buttock area hurt the most. George underwent counseling, treatment with tricyclics and serotonin boosters (Elavil and Celexa), biofeedback, acupuncture, and a graded exercise program. Over the next month, he was weaned off narcotics and prescribed eight Ultram a day for pain. Although George still hurts, his condition has greatly improved.

Controversy arises when a patient has refractory low back pain or joint pain *without* serious radiographic abnormalities. Many of these patients have fibromyalgia, which responds poorly, if at all, to narcotics. Family members sometimes accuse loved ones of having attention-seeking behavior patterns manifesting as chronic musculoskeletal pain. The problem is that some patients can, in fact, physiologically experience truly severe pain with minimal abnormalities in diagnostic tests. On the other hand, some individuals have *psychogenic rheumatism*, where pain complaints are expressed for purposes of secondary gain. The use of narcotics in this setting should be restricted to a pain management center where anesthesiologists, orthopedists, neurosurgeons, and rheumatologists interact with physical therapists and mental health professionals, as well as each other. Chronic musculoskeletal pain patients with psychological problems and only mild to moderately abnormal imaging studies are the most difficult subset of patients doctors encounter. Other medical problems are often overlooked and misdiagnosed. Many of these individuals have had unnecessary or unsuccessful surgeries. In our opinion, their concerns must be taken seriously. A chronic pain patient's problems should be approached respectfully, with the goal of improving physical and psychological function and minimizing the use of narcotics.

Table 16: Managing the pain of osteoarthritis

Topical treatment for local pain
Soothing liniments with camphor or menthol-like substances
Capsaisin
Anti-inflammatory gels with aspirin or NSAIDs

Direct local interventions
Intra-articular steroids
Hyaluronate injections
Joint lavage
Epidural, facet, or sympathetic blocks

Treating inflammatory pain
Aspirin or NSAIDs
Corticosteroids

Treating non-inflammatory, degenerative pain
Aspirin or NSAIDs
Acetaminophen (Tylenol)
Tramodol (Ultram)
Codeine derivatives (e.g., Vicodin)
Propoxyphene derivatives (Darvon)
Pentazocine derivatives (Talwin)
Controlled narcotics (e.g., morphine derivatives)

Surgical removal of source of pain
Arthroscopy
Joint revision, fusion, decompression, or replacement

Managing associated muscle or nerve discomfort
Muscle relaxants (Soma, Norgesic, Parafon, Skelaxin)
Tricyclics (Flexeril, Elavil, Sinequan, Desyrel)
Serotonin boosters (Prozac, Zoloft, Paxil)
Benzodiazepines for spasm (Klonopin, Valium)

Nerve pain blockers (Baclofen, Tegretol, Neurontin)

SUMMARY

Osteoarthritis pain is a major cause of disability and work absences. It stems from many causes, ranging from inflammatory to degenerative, muscular to psychiatric. Various agents are available for each type of pain. Most primary care doctors and musculoskeletal specialists can help pain patients, but chronic, severe musculoskeletal pain usually benefits from a multidisciplinary pain center approach.

21

When Do We Operate?

Doctors approach arthritis patients by steering them into one or more of four general directions. Physical measures, including exercise and rehabilitation, can be recommended. The use of medications—whether prescription, over-the-counter, herbal, or topical—may also be advised. Counseling aspects including general advice, instruction in coping skills, and other psychosocial support systems are made available. And if necessary, an orthopedic referral can be made to consider the possibility of surgery. This chapter will review when and how to consider surgical intervention.

WHO SHOULD BE CONSIDERED FOR SURGERY?

Surgery is not to be approached lightly. Many facets of your medical problems need to be considered. How much pain are you in? How is arthritis altering your lifestyle? What is the extent of the arthritis? Which joints are involved? Are there other medical conditions present? Do you have the time commitment necessary to undergo surgery and its rehabilitation? How much does surgery cost? What kind of rehabilitation activities are associated with the best result? Is there a risk to the surgery? What are the chances it won't work? Will insurance cover it? Will you still have a job to go back to? Who will drive you to the doctor and therapist for the next few weeks? Have medication, physical measures, and counseling approaches accomplished all they can, short of an operation? Orthopedic surgery is not something people just jump into, but it's probably underutilized. (According to one survey, for example, 11% of a community population had X-rays indicating the same or worse arthritis than those who had undergone surgery for it.) If your situation warrants this consideration, read on.

OUTPATIENT PROCEDURES

Advances in technology have enabled the development of "Surgicenters," Where certain procedures can be performed on an outpatient basis. In other words, you get to go home the same day. Some involve minor hand or foot operations, such as removing a bone spur or repairing a torn ligament. Others are discussed below.

Joint lavage

With aging, chronic overuse, and normal wear and tear, our joints may accumulate particles consisting of cartilage debris, crystals, and degradative enzymes. Numerous studies have documented the efficacy of cleaning the joint out. Your orthopedist (and sometimes a rheumatologist) places a trocar (a large bore needle) into the knee, shoulder, or hip and infuses the joint with a salt and water combination. Joint fluid is then drained and the procedure repeated several times. Joint lavage (also known as tidal irrigation) removes the debris and crystals, disrupts intra-articular adhesions, and temporarily cools the joint. Patients often feel better for months to years afterwards. Prospective candidates for joint lavage can be identified by a failure to respond to medications, physical therapy, and injections.

Arthroscopy

Peggy used to ski a lot, but after several ligament and meniscal tears, she stopped. Her knees hurt, but she attributed this to normal stress from the activity. The right knee was much more painful than the left, and her rheumatologist told her that moving it through ranges of motion reminded him of Rice Krispies. An MRI scan documented severe internal derangements along with medial joint-space narrowing. When physical therapy and Aleve failed to improve her condition, the rheumatologist referred her to an orthopedist, who performed arthroscopy. Peggy was amazed that a two-hour outpatient procedure made her largely pain-free within weeks.

Joints can be seen directly through an operating microscope known as an *arthroscope*. During arthroscopy, joint abnormalities can be identified and often repaired. Developed in the 1970s for the knee, arthroscopy is now much more sophisticated and is also used to treat ankles, elbows, shoulders, and wrists. Bone spurs, loose bodies, debris, and crystals can be removed. Tendon and ligament tears and torn menisci can be repaired, the patella can be shaved, and joints lavaged. Arthroscopy is also used diagnostically to obtain biopsies and cultures when the cause of joint disease is not known. The procedure requires a small incision the size of the dime and local anesthesia; and recovery is usually complete within weeks. In rare cases there is a risk that nerves or blood vessels will be cut, but on the whole, arthroscopy is a benign, useful, and successful procedure.

A PRIMER OF ORTHOPEDIC PROCEDURES

There are many different types of joint surgery in addition to joint lavage and arthroscopy. Usually performed on the hip or knee, an *osteotomy* removes or adds a wedge of bone to shift weight bearing. The fusion of two or more bones to decrease pain and promote stability is known as an *arthrodesis*. The wrist and ankle are the most common arthrodesis sites. A total joint replacement is called an *arthroplasty*. For osteoarthritis of the hands or feet, silicone rubber *interposition devices* are placed between the joints. Patients with severe back pain who undergo disc decompression or spinal stenosis surgery have a *laminectomy*. Sometimes bone material is transferred (*grafted*) from one location to another for the purpose of stimulating new bone to fill gaps or holes where deformities exist.

The goal of most surgeries is to preserve or restore a cartilaginous surface. This can be accomplished through joint debridement, resection of subchondral bone to stimulate cartilage formation, or by cartilage or soft tissue grafts. Joint replacement materials can contain plastic, metal, or other synthetic compounds with the goal of promoting a low friction, gliding surface. Orthopedists sometimes try to delay joint replacements by performing osteotomies. Indeed, this buys time. Studies have suggested that remodeling a joint with an osteotomy has a success rate of 70% over one year, 51% over five years, and 30% over ten years time. Knee arthroplasties have a 95% success rate over 15 years, suggesting that they might be appropriate for children. Allowing children to achieve their full growth potential is usually best: replacing a knee at age 20 will have a greater success rate than replacing it at age 10.

JOINT REPLACEMENT (ARTHROPLASTY)

Jo was very nervous about surgery. Her mother died from a blood clot after fracturing her hip, and her best friend has had recurrent infections following ankle operation. When Jo realized that her knee had to be replaced in order to be able to walk, she worked herself into a total panic. She had taken every nonsteroidal available and had failed physical therapy. Three cortisone shots and a course of Synvisc didn't make a bit of difference. Her X-rays showed bone rubbing on bone, and even Percocet provided only temporary relief. Dr. Dabolt walked her through the procedure. She showed Jo a video about knee replacements and gave her a brochure showing her what to expect at every turn. Jo finally consented. She did not panic when prophylactic antibiotics were ordered, or the blood that she donated was returned to her. She remained calm when blood-thinning injections were prescribed and when a huge CPM machine showed up at her bedside after the surgery to provide continuous knee motion. After four days in the acute hospital unit, she was transferred to the rehabilitation floor. Three months later, Jo was pain free and glad she had undergone surgery.

Knee and hip replacements account for 80% of all joint replacement procedures performed in the United States for osteoarthritis. While the surgical success rate is very high, achieving the optimal benefits of an arthroplasty has become an art form, requiring the intricate coordination of internists, rehabilitation specialists and orthopedists. There are important considerations with joint replacement and patients must be carefully screened.

First, a family physician or internist must certify that the patient is medically cleared for surgery. Are there any bleeding or clotting disorders that could interfere? Do any medications need to be withheld because they are associated with increased risks of infection or wound healing? Does the patient have a medical problem such as diabetes or heart failure, which require specific medical management during the stressful period of surgery and its immediate recovery period? Some patients are advised to lose weight before being considered for surgery, as the mechanical stresses on a joint may diminish the probability of a good result. Most patients donate one to three units of their own blood a month or two before surgery, since arthroplasty is associated with some blood loss. Called an *autologous* donation, the blood can be transfused if needed after surgery. Are there anesthesia risks? Shorter, local procedures can be done with local anesthesia (such as nerve blocks or marcaine). Spinal anesthesia is well-tolerated and used for local and less invasive efforts. Arthroplasties are usually performed under general anesthesia. For patients, anesthesia is often the scariest part of undergoing orthopedic surgery, many people fear having someone else control their ability to breathe. Patients are also often uncomfortable for a day or two after surgery. Waking up from anesthesia can involve sweating, nausea, shakes, and a dulled feeling, which fortunately do not last long.

First successfully performed in 1931, arthroplasty has become one of the major treatments for osteoarthritis. Defined as a reconstruction by natural modification, or artificial replacement of a diseased or damaged joint, the availability of arthroplasty became widespread by the 1960s. (An example of a replaced hip joint is shown in Figures 52 and 53). The new joint is constructed with inert metals, a self-curing acrylic resin (methyl methacrylate), and plastic materials. The choice of prosthesis depends on the patient's age and amount of activity the patient will have after surgery. For example, orthopedists tend to use cementless hip replacements for younger patients who want to resume athletic activity. Joint replacements for the ankle, shoulder, and elbow are also available, but are used much less frequently and do not work as well.

Individuals who undergo hip or knee replacements are usually in the hospital for three to seven days. During this time they are often prescribed blood-thinning medicines, antibiotics, and narcotic pain preparations.

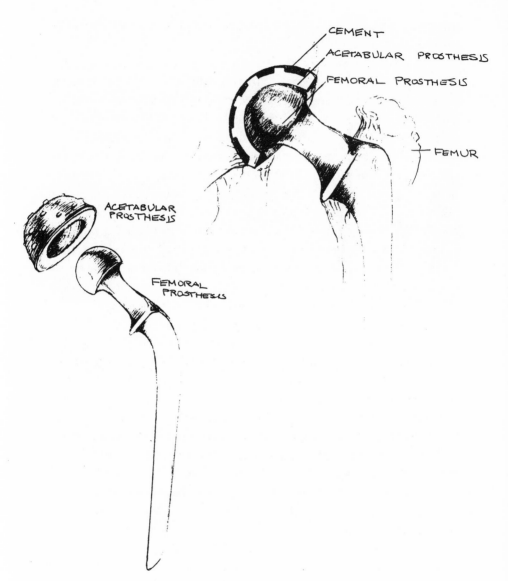

CEMENT

ACETABULAR PROSTHESIS

FEMORAL PROSTHESIS

FEMUR

ACETABULAR PROSTHESIS

FEMORAL PROSTHESIS

FIG. 52   *Hip replacement surgery*

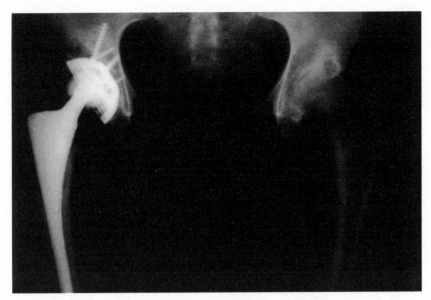

FIG. 53   *X-ray of a surgically replaced hip*

Mobilization and rehabilitation occur when they are medically stable. Knee patients are usually given continuous passive motion (CPM), a device which prevents adhesions and scars from forming. Many patients are transferred to a rehabilitation hospital setting for an additional week or two. During this time, they receive intensive physical and occupational therapy for two to six hours a day. Advice is provided for. For example, hip replacement patients are told to avoid having their knees higher than their hips, crossing their legs, bending, twisting, or leaning forward while seated.

What can go wrong?

Sometimes patients ask us, "What's the worst that can happen?" The most common complications of arthroplasty are shaft fracture (in up to 10% of cases) dislocation (1–5%), nerve damage (1–3%), pulmonary embolus (1–4%), and death (one case per thousand). The long-term side effects include deep infection (a 1% rate over 10 years), and loosening of the prosthesis (10% over 10 years). Some patients need a second procedure five to fifteen years later, to deal with loosening or to put in a second joint. Despite these risks, orthopedic surgery is an overwhelmingly safe, effective and function promoting endeavor.

SUMMARY

Surgery has clearly come a long way. We can now perform arthroscopy and replace just about any joint. Total joint replacements of the hip and knee can last over 20 years. Bone transplantation, cartilage grafts, sophisticated bone reconstruction procedures, and gene therapies are in their infancy. Better plastic materials and metal alloys are becoming available all the time.

22

Alternative Therapies

Do They Work?

Orthodox medicine has not found an answer to your complaint.
However, luckily for you, I happen to be a quack.
                                      —Charles Richter, from his cartoon

As we have mentioned, there is no real cure for osteoarthritis, and some of the interventions practitioners recommend have complications or undesirable side effects. It is logical that many individuals seek out other options. Alternative or complementary approaches refer to a broad range of therapies or health care practices not generally learned in conventional medical training or used in general medical practice. In 1997, Americans spent $15 billion in out-of-pocket expenses on alternative therapies. Some of these approaches must work, or people would not continue to waste their money. This section will attempt to place complementary therapies in perspective.

WHO PROVIDES OR PRESCRIBES ALTERNATIVE THERAPIES?

Any physician, allied health professional or alternative practioner can advocate or prescribe complementary regimens, and patients can undergo these approaches without seeing a musculoskeletal practitioner. In certain countries (e.g., China), what we consider to be alternative therapies are the remedies most commonly prescribed by mainstream physicians.

DIETARY SUPPLEMENTS

As discussed in Chapter 17, approved arthritis medications must adhere to very high standards in order to receive the endorsement of the Food and Drug Administration. Although many complementary remedies are really drugs, most are considered to be food supplements or *nutriceuticals* by the United States government. As a consequence, they are available over-the-counter and are rarely tested in the strict environment that prescription drugs are. Labelling can be misleading, and claims of efficacy or indications for use don't have be proven. In a 1999 sampling of several health food store versions of 25 mg dehydroepiandrosterone tablets (DHEA), the content actually ranged from zero to 50 milligrams. Bioavailability is also a variable. There is no assurance that the coating or preservative in an alternative agent allows it to be absorbed to take in the number of milligrams on the label. The coatings and preservatives may also cause adverse reactions, and contain food dyes that are not related to the food supplement itself. What follows is a review of these dietary supplements, based on the best information available.

Chondroitin sulfate/glucosamine

As a result of Dr. Jason Theodasakis' best selling book *The Arthritis Cure*, combinations of chondroitin sulfate/glucosamine have become the most popular dietary supplements used in managing joint pains. This agent does have positive effects, although it is not a cure.

Chondroitin sulfate is a sugar that is part of the cartilage-proteoglycan complex, and gives articular cartilage its ability to absorb shock. When putting weight on the knee joint, chondroitin helps push joint fluid out. When taking weight off the knee, chondroitin helps bring the fluid back in. In osteoarthritis, the amount of chondroitin in articular cartilage goes down, and with it the shock-absorbing ability of cartilage decreases.

The chondroitin sulfate easily obtained today at health food stores is usually chemically synthesized, and often sold with glucosamine. These two sugars are part of the articular cartilage. Since the amount of these sugars decreases with osteoarthritis and articular cartilage destruction, it is suggested that if you take some of these sugars by mouth, they will move through the bloodstream to the cartilage and help it regain its shock-absorbing capacity. If your osteoarthritic knee has more shock absorption capacity, then the pain may decrease or go away.

Glucosamine, either with hydrochloride or sulfate, and with and without chondroitin sulfate, is also now frequently prescribed. Like chondroitin, glucosamine is a sugar that is part of cartilage and appears to reduce joint pain by as yet undefined mechanisms.

Dozens of small studies have been done to evaluate chondroitin. A definitive study has been funded by the National Institutes of Health, the results of which will not be known for several years. Available information tends to show that these compounds reduce pain about the same amount as nonsteroidals, over a period of several months. Chondroitin sulfate/glucosamine improves mild-to-moderate osteoarthritis of the knee and hand as well as general aches and pains, but it has little effect on severe osteoarthritis. Glucosamine may prevent joint deterioration, and can be as effective as ibuprofen. How these complex sugars actually work, however, is speculative. The usual dose of glucosamine is 1500 mg a day in divided doses. Patients usually don't notice a difference for two to three months. Since these preparations cost more than over-the-counter nonsteroidals, and insurance does not pay for them, we recommend that you review the internet site www.Dr.theo.com in order to assess which preparations have the best bioavailability.

Treatment with these compounds appears to be free of any serious or significant side effects, but safety issues have not been adequately studied. Chondroitin is structurally similar to the blood-thinning preparation heparin, and in high doses some patients may experience some bleeding. Patients also occasionally complain of nausea. Glucosamine can increase blood sugar in animals (and maybe in humans), and is not recommended in individuals who are allergic to shellfish. Also, chondroitin sulfate and glucosamine are often combined with a variety of other substances. Show your physician the label of the product you are taking.

OTHER ALTERNATIVE PREPARATIONS

It is important that you consult your health care provider before taking any of these treatments. The efficacies and toxicities listed in the discussion below are based on small-scale studies and should not be regarded as definitive.

Avacado/soybean oils or unsaponifiables (ASU) have been hypothesized to stimulate cartilage production, but this has not been shown in clinical studies. It may improve pain and function in patients with knee or hip osteoarthritis, and appears to be free of any serious side effects.

Boron helps with calcium and magnesium metabolism, and has been studied in cases of osteoarthritis, rheumatoid arthritis, and osteoporosis. Boron is found in many fruits, vegetables, and nuts and is a component of many multivitamin formulations. A single small osteoarthritis study suggested that it may improve pain and decrease joint swelling. High doses of boron (above 3 mg a day) can raise estrogen levels.

Boswellia (frankincense, salai guggal) is derived from a tree in Asia. In India, tree gum from Boswellia serrata is used to treat arthritic pain. Some studies suggest that it has anti-inflammatory properties, while others found that it did not. It may have modest anti-arthritic efficacy. Boswellia is usually sold in combination with other ingredients, but as the gum extract oleoresin, it is taken in doses of 150 mg three times a day.

Curcumin (tumeric) is a root found in India and China, where it is used to treat joint pains. Often combined with boswella, zinc, ginger or aswangandha, it has some anti-inflammatory properties. Taken in doses of 400 mg up to three times a day, curcumin is not recommended during pregnancy or in individuals who have gall stones.

Capsaican cayenne, comes from the seeds and membranes of nightshade. Cayenne (red pepper) is extracted from seeds and membranes of the nightshade family of plants. This agent blocks release of substance P (a pain mediator). It is applied as a cream, multiple times a day (Chapter 19).

Fish oils contain omega-3 fatty acids (eicosapentaenoic acid and docasohexaemoic acid), which reduce joint inflammation in laboratory studies and are clinically beneficial in rheumatoid arthritis and mice with lupus. They can lower cholesterol levels, but can also thin the blood. There are some suggestions from the rheumatoid arthritis studies that coexisting osteoarthritis also improved.

Ginger is a root commonly used in Asian cooking. Taken in tea, capsules, or as a hot compress, it may reduce osteoarthritis pain and inflammation. In larger doses it can upset the stomach and increase the risk of bleeding.

Methyl sulfonyl methane (MSM) is derived from a sulfur compound broken down by dimethyl sulfoxide (DMSO). DMSO is a by-product of wood processing and a chemical used in paint thinner and antifreeze. Heavily promoted by a well-known Hollywood actor, there are no peer-reviewed studies of its use in osteoarthritis.

SAMe (S-adenosylmethionine) is a natural compound produced when the amino acid methionine combines with a cellular fuel known as ATP.

Table 17: Daily recommended doses for selected vitamins and minerals

Vitamins or minerals	Daily recommended dose
Vitamin A	2500 IU/day for women, 5000 IU/day for men
Vitamin B3 (niacinamide)	10–25 mg/day
Vitamin B5 (panthothentic acid)	250 mg/day
Vitamin B12	Multivitamin containing B12
Vitamin C	500–1000 mg/day
Vitamin D	400–800 IU/day
Vitamin E	400–600 IU/day
Calcium	1000–1500 mg/day
Folic acid	1 mg/day

It is widely used in Europe to manage depression. Increasing ATP levels may also decrease joint pain, especially when combined with folic acid. The dose used is 200 mg to 400 mg three times a day.

St John's Wort is a small yellow flower grown throughout the United States and Europe. Containing hypericin and hyperforin, it increases serotonin levels in the brain and is widely used in Europe as "nature's Prozac" to treat depression. It has no known effects on arthritis, but patients given serotonin-boosting antidepressants often have less joint pain.

Stinging nettle is a herb that induces stinging pain, and possibly has anti-inflammatory effects when applied to the skin. In one study, it was effective as nonsteroidal anti-inflammatory agents in treating osteoarthritis pain and joint stiffness.

Are vitamins or minerals helpful?

Free radicals are present throughout our body, and an excess of them can result in tissue destruction, aging, and cancer. They are destroyed by antioxidants, which include vitamins C, E, beta carotene flavinoids, lutein, and the mineral selenium. Epidemiologic studies from the southern United States have suggested that a diet high in antioxidants decreases the risk for developing osteoarthritis. One survey found that vitamins C, D, and E reduced the risk for developing knee osteoarthritis. Another survey, however, suggested that beta-carotene (vitamin A) increases the risk for evolving knee osteoarthritis. We recommend that all arthritis patients take a multivitamin product on a regular basis; the specific suggested ingredients are shown in Table 17.

SUMMARY

Though many alternative remedies, herbs, vitamins, and minerals are thought to help osteoarthritis, only a few have been studied in a rigorous, double-blind, placebo-controlled fashion. There is some evidence that glucosamine/chondroitin sulfate combinations and many remedies used in Europe and Asia have some anti-arthritis properties, and that vitamins and minerals may help prevent bone and tissue destruction. Unfortunately, these treatments are not standardized, and their use should be coordinated with a musculoskeletal health care specialist to prevent adverse reactions.

23

I Have Osteoarthritis

Who Should I Go to for Treatment?

Medicine should be practiced as a form of friendship.
　　　　　　　　　　　　　　—Léon Bernard, born 1875

Twenty-three million people in the United States have osteoarthritis. Most have mild or localized symptoms, some have none. Other patients are crippled by the degenerative process. Many different physicians and allied health professionals manage osteoarthritis. Sometimes the cast of characters can be confusing. Who should be consulted and what is the optimal process?

PHYSICIANS

Physicians are medical doctors who have completed four years of medical school after an undergraduate education. In order to be licensed to practice in the United States, all physicians have to complete a postgraduate year or internship, and pass the National Board Exams. A physician who stops their training at this point is a general practitioner, or GP. A GP usually has had, at best, a few weeks of training in arthritis.

Following internship (also known as a first-year residency), about 90% of United States medical school graduates complete two additional years of training, or residency. Residency programs are offered in internal medicine, surgery, family practice, pediatrics, obstetrics-gynecology, radiology, and psychiatry, among other fields. Concerning the manage-

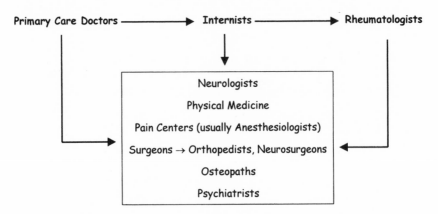

FIG. 54 *Health care professionals who manage osteoarthritis referral patterns*

ment of arthritis, family practice physicians have one to two months of training in orthopedics and rheumatology, and treat mild strains or traumas as well as uncomplicated osteoarthritis with acetaminophen, NSAIDs, and physical measures. They refer more complicated cases to internists, rheumatologists, or orthopedists. Internists have one to two months of training in rheumatology but none in orthopedics. Osteoarthritis generally takes up about 10% of an internist's time, and 10% of their patients are referred to rheumatologists or orthopedists. (See Figure 54).

What is a rheumatologist?

Rheumatologists are internists who have completed an additional two to three years of subspecialty training covering aspects of musculoskeletal complaints and disorders of the immune system. They diagnose symptoms as a specific type of arthritis, and order diagnostic studies, prescribe medication, deal with potential drug interactions, inject joints, and supervise rehabilitation programs. There are 5,000 practicing rheumatologists in the United States, representing 1% of all physicians. Difficult diagnostic challenges and complicated therapeutic approaches are usually directed to a rheumatologist. Some rheumatologists also act as a family or primary care doctor; others function strictly as consultants.

What is an orthopedist?

Orthopedists are physicians who have completed part or all of a surgical internship and residency and three years of specialty training. They specialize in the treatment of fractures, bone tumors, and musculoskeletal complaints, and perform joint replacements. They can diagnose most musculoskeletal conditions, but generally only work with patients who need injections or surgery. There are approximately 40,000 orthopedists in the United States.

What is a physiatrist?

Also known as a rehabilitation medicine physician, physiatrists enter a physical medicine residency after their internship. Often hospital-based, physiatrists supervise recovery and rehabilitation programs for patients who need intensive, coordinated care for problems such as strokes, complicated wounds, and amputations. They frequently work as part of a team with physical therapists, occupational therapists, speech pathologists, psychologists, and other allied health professionals. Osteoarthritis patients might find themselves under a physiatrist's care while being assisted in their recovery from major joint replacement surgery. About 3,000 physicians in the United States are physiatrists.

What is a neurologist?

After a medical internship, some doctors enter a three-year residency program in neurology. Neurologists do not practice primary care; they diagnose and medically treat strokes, headaches, seizures, and neuropathies in concert with internists. Patients with osteoarthritis might consult a neurologist to rule out a spinal nerve injury, impingement, or radiculopathy, to evaluate symptoms of numbness or tingling, or undergo an electrical study such as an EMG or nerve conduction.

What is a neurosurgeon?

After one to two years of a surgical residency, some doctors enroll in a three to four year program to be trained as neurosurgeons. They operate on the brain, spinal cord, and peripheral nerves. Frequently, orthopedists work with and assist neurosurgeons (and vice versa) when performing complicated spinal operations. Osteoarthritis patients with a herniated disc or spinal stenosis may be referred to a neurosurgeon.

What is an anesthesiologist?

Anesthesiologists are physicians who put patients to sleep so that they can undergo surgery. In recent years anesthesiologists have branched out and play a leading role in coordinating pain management. In this context, an osteoarthritis patient might consult an anesthesiologist for an epidural or nerve block to treat a herniated disc or spinal stenosis, to receive a complicated injection (into a facet joint, for example), or to manage chronic arthritis pain.

What is an osteopath?

Although osteopaths have a title of D.O. (doctor of osteopathy) rather than M.D. (medical doctor), in the United States they are considered equal to M.D.s and are allowed to perform surgery and prescribe medicine. In the United States graduates of osteopathic medical schools undertake osteopathic medical training which is almost identical to a school that trains M.D.s. Most of them go on to internships or residency programs run by M.D.s and not osteopathic institutions. Historically, osteopaths had specialized skills in spinal manipulation in the management of musculoskeletal conditions, but today fewer than 20% practice manipulation. The majority of D.O.s engage in primary care, internal medicine, or family practice.

DOCTORS FOR SPECIFIC BODY REGIONS

Dentists and *podiatrists* are allowed to perform surgery and prescribe medication for conditions affecting the oral cavity and foot and ankle, respectively. They have at least four years of professional training after completing college. Patients with temporomandibular osteoarthritis might consult dentists who are TMJ specialists. Podiatrists can manage most arthritic conditions of the foot and ankle, and make footwear recommendations. *Chiropractors* complete four years of training after high school. They are well-versed in physical medicine modalities, especially spinal manipulation, which is helpful to some osteoarthritis patients. Chiropractors cannot prescribe medication or perform surgery.

WHICH ALLIED HEALTH PROFESSIONALS ASSIST OSTEOARTHRITIS PATIENTS?

In a doctor's office there may be times when a *physician's assistant* or *nurse practitioner* are the first health professional you see. Although their responsibilities are dictated by differing state laws, PAs and NPs can usually write prescriptions for certain arthritis medications. PAs often have a paramedic or armed forces medic background, and NPs are registered nurses (RNs) with advanced training. All of their notes must be discussed with and reviewed by a physician.

Physical therapists undergo a three-year training program after at least two years of college. They are frequently called upon to assist osteoarthritis patients by using methods to improve function and decrease pain. These include massage, heat, ice, electrical stimulation, manipulation, myofascial release, posture and gait training, and exercise regimens. *Occupational therapists* have similar training to physical therapists and, through an "Activities of Daily Living" evaluation, instruct patients in the principles of energy conservation and joint protection. Osteoarthritis patients with back pain, for example, benefit from an occupational therapy evaluation of their workstation. A lumbar band with a high desk counter might be recommended. Occupational therapists are also skilled in the art of splinting and bracing, evaluating and preventing repetitive strains at a computer desk, and recommending assistive devices. Additional needs of osteoarthritis patients may be serviced by *psychologists, counselors, clergy,* or *social workers* who can advise them of available community resources, as well as providing emotional support.

WHAT ALTERNATIVE PRACTITIONERS MANAGE OSTEOARTHRITIS?

Many patients don't want to take medication. Others prefer a more "natural" approach. Some seek a way to avoid recommended surgery. Many physicians encourage or steer patients towards complementary or alternative medicine remedies. (We reviewed some of these approaches in chapter 22). Alternative practitioners are often physicians, osteopaths, or chiropractors, but view themselves as "healers" using different approaches. *Acupuncturists* (who are usually not physicians) mobilize one's chi, or energizing life force energy, which flows throughout the body. By putting specialized needles in specified points along the meridians, some patients experience pain relief. *Homeopaths* (most of whom are M.D.s) work on the principle that administering infinitesimally small doses of harmful substances promotes protection against them. Used for over two hundred years, homeopathic medicines usually consist of small amounts of plant extracts. Several thousand doctors in the United States have taken courses in homeopathy, although the major tenets of the approach remain controversial. Homeopathic preparations, some of which might help osteoarthritis, are readily available without prescription.

WHAT'S THE BOTTOM LINE? WHO SHOULD I GO TO?

Patients with a musculoskeletal complaint that is thought to be osteoarthritis should first consult their primary care physician. Most of the time, no further consultation is necessary. Laboratory tests, imaging evaluations, medication, or physical remedies can be requested or prescribed. When appropriate, a subspecialist, allied health professional, dentist, or podiatrist may be consulted. Most patients with problematic osteoarthritis are evaluated by rheumatologists and/or orthopedists. If you decide to seek out a musculoskeletal consultation on your own, advise your primary care doctor that you are doing so in order to keep a record, monitor results, coordinate therapy, or make sure that proposed interventions require more rigorous consideration and consultation.

24

Special Cases

Osteoarthritis from Childhood Events and During Pregnancy

Parents learn a lot from their children about coping with life.
—Muriel Spark

We've been asked at times if children can develop osteoarthritis. After all, most people think of osteoarthritis as a disease of aging. Although there are forms of arthritis evident in childhood, such as juvenile rheumatoid arthritis, juvenile spondylitis, lupus, and Kawasaki's disease, osteoarthritis, per se, is not present in children. Nevertheless, certain formative features of bone which become evident during growth ensure or greatly increase the risk of osteoarthritis in later life. These will be reviewed here, along with a consideration of what happens when pregnancy occurs in osteoarthritis patients.

CAN PEOPLE BE BORN WITH OSTEOARTHRITIS OR DEVELOP IT AS CHILDREN?

Collagen is a form of loose connective tissue that is responsible for certain aspects of bone formation. Hyaline cartilage consists of large amounts of Type II collagen. Gene mutations have been described in families that result in the underproduction of Type II collagen. These individuals tend to develop early osteoarthritis with an onset during adolescence, and it tends to involve weight-bearing joints. Trying to identify the genes that can program the body towards developing osteoarthritis is the focus of intense scrutiny. However, the going has not been easy. It appears that there are many different gene markers involved in osteoarthritis predisposition. Some are point mutations, deletions, or substitutions, and they tend to occur in isolated families.

Dysplasia of the epiphysis (the bone growth plate) associated with abnormalities of the precursor of Type II collagen genes results in deformed bones. This can lead to precocious classical osteoarthritis, and variants where eburnation is absent or the cartilage is shaggy in appearance. For example, these situations may occur in individuals who have dislocated hips at birth, certain types of dwarfism, and hypermobility syndromes. In the latter, joints are prone to dislocation, and tendons or ligaments tend to rupture with trivial trauma. Hyperelasticity states associated with accelerated osteoarthritis include Ehlers-Danlos syndrome, osteogenesis imperfecti or Marfan's syndrome.

DEVELOPMENTAL EVENTS WHICH PREDISPOSE TOWARD OSTEOARTHRITIS

Four types of events lead to premature osteoarthritis. They include localized problems, mechanical irregularities, epiphyseal bone dysplasia, and trauma.

Localized events

The overwhelming majority of local events resulting in early osteoarthritis occur in the hip and involves mechanical defects. Congenital dislocation of the hip does not result in osteoarthritis if it is definitively corrected before the age of six.

Henry told his father that his hip hurt. Since he was only eight years old and had not injured anything, his parents did not take it seriously. After a few weeks, he began to limp. Henry was taken to the pediatrician, who found an abnormal hip X-ray. An MRI suggested Legg-Calve-Perthes disease. An orthopedist was consulted, who advised that Henry would ultimately need surgery. He also told him to minimize weight-bearing. Henry got upset that he couldn't play baseball, and his schoolwork suffered. Casting the hip in abduction was discussed, but the family decided against it, since Henry's fragile emotional state could not take any more setbacks. Finally, Henry underwent a hip replacement. Even though he knew it would have to be revised and redone on several occasions over his lifetime, Henry no longer needed home schooling and was able to participate in most activities.

Legg-Calve-Perthes disease is a condition similar to *osteonecrosis* or *avascular necrosis,* where dead bone is found in the hip. It occurs between the ages of four and nine, with the cases in boys outnumbering those in girls by 4 to 1. Most patients have a painful limp. X-rays or imaging studies suggest effusion, or fluid in the hip. Occasionally, the child may complain of knee pain, when, in fact, this perception is referred pain from the hip. Mild cases are treated with nonsteroidal anti-inflammatory drugs. Abduction casting for periods of a year or more are brutal and psychologically devastating, but may delay or prevent surgery. Surgery is usually ultimately needed in nearly all patients, but there is some flexibility in timing. Failure to perform surgery during childhood, however, leads to a certainty of osteoarthritis of the hip by early adulthood. What should a parent do? An orthopedist, in consultation with the pediatrician, usually provide a variety of options.

Mechanical defects

Tall, thin children are susceptible to *slipped capital femoral epiphysis,* where the growth plate moves down from the rest of the bone. It may require surgical correction and is associated with early-onset osteoarthritis.

A growing child experiences changes in expanding structures such as tendons, ligaments, bony growth, and closure of the epiphyses. Infrequently, one extremity may grow disproportionate to the other, or ligaments and tendons may produce abnormalities when walking. Examples of this, which can lead to premature osteoarthritis, include leg length discrepancies, turning in or out of the knee while walking (being knock-kneed or pigeon-toed), or scoliosis. In the case of scoliosis, small curvatures of the spine become accentuated during growth, which eventually lead to osteoarthritis changes in the spine by midlife. Pediatricians usually screen for pronated feet in young children or failure to develop arches by adolescence, which also lead to early osteoarthritis and foot pain. During a child's annual examination, an astute pediatrician who carefully monitors growth and development landmarks can usually identify these mechanical problems. Preventive measures include splinting, bracing, exercises, and occasionally surgery.

Some children have very lax ligaments or tendons and can extend their elbows or knees beyond a straight line of 180 degrees, or touch their forearms with the thumbs, or seemingly twirl their ankles around. While a host of genetic disorders associated with collagen defects can cause this (Ehlers-Danlos syndrome, Marfan's, pseudoxanthoma elasticum, etc.), the overwhelming majority of these children are completely healthy. Known as *benign hypermobility syndrome*, at first these children seem to be very promising in ballet, gymnastics, or similar endeavors, only to rupture a ligament or tendon at a critically inopportune moment. The treatment of benign hypermobility involves providing mechanical support to the supporting structures of joints, avoiding excessive athletic activities, and muscle strengthening (especially the quadriceps). Patients with benign hypermobility syndrome who have had several dislocations, fractures, or ruptures during their formative years almost always develop premature osteoarthritis.

Bone dysplasias

As noted in Chapter 4, there are several structural regions of bone structure and growth known as the epiphysis, metaphysis and diaphysis. Abnormal developmental changes in these regions are *dysplasias*. Abnormalities of the metaphysis or diaphysis produce different types of dwarfism and metabolic disorders. As a child matures, their growth plate (the epiphysis) closes and becomes normal adult bone (see Figure 55). This may occur as early as age four in certain bone structure regions and as late as age twenty-three in the coccyx or tail bone. A variety of disorders lead to epiphyseal dysplasias. Premature closure of the epiphysis can result from juvenile rheumatoid arthritis or systemic lupus, with resulting shortened adult stature. Thyroid disorders, corticosteroids, sickle cell anemia, and kidney failure also are associated with epiphyseal problems. Fragmentation of the epiphysis in the bones produces premature osteoarthritis. This is usually the result of a trauma. For example, stress fractures associated with excessive exercise in ballet, gymnastics, running, marching, or jumping can fragment the epiphysis.

Other traumatic conditions known to cause early onset osteoarthritis stem from childhood events that lead to avascular necrosis; not enough oxygen gets into the bone, and it dies. These conditions include Kohler's disease (avascular necrosis of the tarsal-navicular joint), Freiberg's disease (involving the metatarsal head of the toes), and Kienbock's (affecting the lunate in the wrist). There is also Scheurmann's disease (when an adolescent herniates a disc due to a defective ring such as epiphysis of the vertebrae), Osgood-Schlatter's syndrome (a partial avulsion of the patellar tendon, leading to a bony growth on the tibial tubercle), and calcaneal apophysitis (from avulsion of the Achilles tendon).

PREVENTIVE STRATEGIES

Parents should do everything they can to prevent their child from evolving a condition which could plague them for most of their adult life. The best preventive strategy includes a yearly check-up with the pediatrician. If your child is engaged in competitive or rigorous sports activities, have a talk with the trainer or sports medicine doctor to minimize harm that may come from these efforts. Should you have your son or daughter take an Advil or ice a joint before exercising? Are there supportive devices, taping, or bandaging which can obviate problems and diminish risks? If your child has a limp, postural problem, or appears to walk oddly, make sure that a pediatric orthopedist or rheumatologist performs a clinical evaluation. Children should be educated about the activities they are involved in, how to take care of themselves, what to do if they are injured, and what the consequences are of being noncompliant.

PREGNANCY CONSIDERATIONS

If, as a child, any of the considerations listed above applied to you, it is likely that you will already have osteoarthritis by the time of pregnancy. Many women with painful Hebreden's or Bouchard's nodes in the hands also experience discomfort during pregnancy. What happens to osteoarthritis during a pregnancy? Most pregnant women notice little difference, other than difficulty getting around in the third trimester.

What medicines are safe to take for arthritis during pregnancy?

There are only two safe treatment approaches for a pregnant woman. Acetaminophen (Tylenol) helps non inflammatory osteoarthritis, and can be used in doses up to eight 325 mg tablets a day. Nonsteroidal anti-inflammatory agents and aspirin are not advised during pregnancy, except for occasional use. Their use can delay closure of a pathway in the fetal heart. Known as the *ductus arteriosis*, this heart canal must close before delivery in order to prevent cardiac problems in the newborn. Inflammatory osteoarthritis is best managed by local injections of corticosteroids. Steroids are a natural body hormone made by the adrenal gland, and their occasional use poses no problems for a pregnant woman. In rare instances, oral corticosteroids may be needed for a short period of time. Some herbs and alternative therapies may be harmful in pregnancy. Ask your doctor before taking any of these preparations.

One type of arthritis known to develop during pregnancy is *transient osteoporosis of pregnancy*. This rare condition almost always occurs in the hip. It produces a dull, throbbing ache in the hip region, and is associated with a high blood sedimentation rate and an effusion that can be seen in an ultrasound. Diagnosed using X-ray (with the fetus shielded), transient osteoporosis of pregnancy is usually a benign condition which resolves itself within a few weeks of delivery. In rare cases, it leads to fractures or premature osteoarthritic changes in the hip region.

SUMMARY

Although children can develop various types of arthritis, osteoarthritis is not one of them. However, childhood activities and growth anomalies can lead to its development during early adulthood. The pediatrician and sports trainer represent the first lines of prevention and detection, along with educating our youth about the implications of vigorous activity when their bones and growth plates are not fully matured. Pregnant women may have osteoarthrtis, which temporarily limits their choice of medication.

Part VI

OUTCOME AND FUTURE DIRECTIONS

If you look over a list of medicinal recipes in vogue in the last century, how foolish and useless they are seen to be! And yet we use equally absurd ones with faith today.
 —Henry David Thoreau, *Journal* (1860)

This final section begins with a discussion of what happens to the 23 million Americans with osteoarthritis. Can they work or do they qualify for disability benefits (chapter 25)? What is the long-term prognosis for patients with osteoarthritis (chapter 26)? And then there is the most exciting part of the book—and the section we most enjoyed writing: the future. Advances in biochemistry, genetics, pharmacology, and physiology have resulted in the years 2000-2010 being declared the "Bone and Joint Decade" by the World Health Organization. Chapter 27 will provide the reader with a sneak preview of exciting advances the public will be learning about.

25

Can or Should I Work?

Every man's task is his life preserver.
                —Ralph Waldo Emerson, "Worship" (1860)

Though seemingly as benign as the common cold, osteoarthritis is a public health menace to be reckoned with. Causing over 700,000 hospitalizations per year in the United States, the disease and its related health care visits lead to 68 million days of missed work, annually. Another 1.5 billion dollars are lost due to restricted work activities, making osteoarthritis the second most common cause of disability in the United States. These figures depend on how the definition of "disability" is used, and how work abilities are assessed. A survey of patients with X-ray findings indicating osteoarthritis found that 30% had symptoms only, 20% felt it was a "significant health problem," 7% had some restricted activity or form of disability, and only 0.5% had a severe disability. Nevertheless, if 60 million Americans have the criteria on X-ray consistent with osteoarthritis, this translates to 4.2 million people with some disability, and 300,000 people with severe disability. This chapter will address disability issues.

WHAT IS DISABILITY?

According to the World Health Organization, disability is "a restriction or lack of ability to perform an activity in a manner within the range considered normal due to impairments or handicaps." An impairment is an anatomic, physiologic, or psychological loss. This includes pain from work activities (e.g., heavy lifting), emotional stress (having a job such as customer service representative for an airline), or muscle dysfunction (e.g., cerebral palsy). A handicap is a job limitation or something that cannot be done (because of blindness, deafness, etc.).

The science of quantitating or assessing disability is inexact, and subject to many variables and concerns. For instance, disability is not purely biologic; it can be altered by coping and adaptation strategies. Efforts to manage work disabilities consider issues such as age, sex, level of education, psychological profile, past attainments, motivation, retraining prospects, work-related self-esteem, motivation, stress, fatigue, personal value systems, and availability of financial compensation. Disability analysts usually depend on four measures to evaluate work performance: ability to perform functional activities, the activities of daily living (ADL) assessment, the presence of selected impairments, and the use of assistive aids. Again, these evaluations are subject to numerous considerations. For example, people who encounter functional limitations are not disabled if society is able to accommodate alternative methods of functioning, such as providing a wheelchair and ramps.

An ADL evaluation is usually performed by an occupational therapist and specifically looks at eleven domains: locomotion (e.g., the ability to walk or climb stairs): transportation (whether a patient is able to drive or take a bus); transfers (sitting-to-stand, moving on and off a toilet seat); personal hygiene (grooming); dressing (e.g., putting on shoes); feeding (the ability to eat and take pills); environment (e.g., light, room temperature); communication (the ability to speak and write); recreational activities; homemaking (activities such as shopping and cleaning house); and work (lifting, pulling, or other activities). The ADL and other evaluations can be easily biased by the specialist performing the assessment. For example, consider the implications of answering a question worded three different ways: Do you tie your own shoes? Can you tie your own shoes? If you had to, could you tie your own shoes?

WHAT ARE THE PREDICTORS OF WORK DISABILITY?

Taking all of the above factors into account, how does this translate into the ability to hold a job? The four major predictive areas deal with work autonomy (the control you have over your work pace and activities), work-based social factors (cooperation with bosses and co-workers, attitudes towards disability, getting to and from work), disease factors (restricted bodily functioning, physical barriers to work), and home/personal factors (your level of education, depression, and amount of family support).

WORK DISABILITY IN OSTEOARTHRITIS

The most common reasons why patients with osteoarthritis are unable to work are pain, muscle weakness, joint impairments, and functional limitations. These vary depending on the joint studied. The overwhelming majority of osteoarthritis patients on disability have abnormalities in the hip, knee, or back.

A so-called "index of function" was once devised based on the presence of tenderness, swelling, decreased range of motion, crepitus, and deformity. This turned out to be totally useless unless age, sex, education, income, personal and health habits, motivation, social support, physical environment, anxiety, depression, and coping style were factored into the equation. For instance, among disabled women with osteoarthritis, there is a higher frequency of divorce, and subjects are more likely to receive welfare payments.

Different restrictions are unique to different joints. For example, the inability to flex the knee to 70 degrees causes difficulty walking, transferring to a toilet seat, walking up and down stairs, or getting in or out of a bathtub. A variety of "co-morbidities" also exist. In other words, osteoarthritis of the knee in individuals over the age of 65 is more frequently associated with disability if one also has heart disease, lung disease, or is overweight.

WHO IS ELIGIBLE FOR DISABILITY IN THE UNITED STATES?

All states have a form of workers' compensation, which is a type of disability insurance. Most large employers also provide disability insurance, and many self-employed individuals pay for their own policy. Patients with a disability can be determined to be "permanently, and totally disabled," and thus potentially eligible for Social Security and Medicare health benefits. Other classifications include being "permanently, partially disabled," whereby vocational rehabilitation, occupational therapy, and psychological or workstation evaluations can address impairments or handicaps to optimize employment retraining possibilities. A classification of "temporary, partial disability" allows one to work with restrictions (e.g., not lifting more than 10 pounds) while treatment is in progress. This may also involve a leave of absence from employment while undergoing treatment.

Subjective factors of disability include symptoms such as pain or fatigue, while objective factors of disability are physical signs such as a heart murmur or swollen joint. One can be disabled from a particular category of work and granted disability even if employment is ongoing in a different work category. Work categories are rated as sedentary, light work, light medium work, medium work, heavy work, or very heavy work, each defined by how much exertion is used over a time interval. Another consideration is given to repetitive motions such as bending, squatting, walking up stairs, and squeezing, as well as environmental temperature or the operation of heavy equipment. The Americans with Disabilities Act protects individuals from job discrimination by requiring companies with more than 15 employees to make reasonable accommodations for people with disabilities and chronic illnesses.

WHAT ARE THE DEFINITIONS FOR TOTAL DISABILITY FOR OSTEOARTHRITIS?

The following is a condensed Listing of Impairments put together by the United States Government and published as *Disability Evaluation under Social Security*. Sections applicable to osteoarthritis, which allow for Social Security disability and Medicare health benefits, are detailed below.

1.00 Musculoskeletal System

A. Loss of function may be due to amputation or deformity. Pain may be an important factor in causing functional loss, but it must be associated with relevant abnormal signs or laboratory findings . . .

B. Disorders of the spine, associated with vertebrogenic disorders as in 1.05C, result in impairment because of distortion of the bony and ligamentous architecture of the spine or impingement of a herniated nucleus pulpous or bulging annulus on a nerve root. Impairment caused by such abnormalities usually improves with time or responds to treatment. Appropriate physical findings must be shown to persist on repeated examinations despite therapy for a reasonable presumption to be made that severe impairment will last for a continuous period of 12 months. This may occur in cases with unsuccessful prior surgical treatment . . .

C. After maximum benefit from surgical therapy has been achieved in situations involving fractures of an upper extremity or injuries to the soft tissues of a lower or upper extremity . . .

> (i) Effects of obesity. Obesity . . . is often associated with disturbance of the musculoskeletal system and disturbance of this system can be a major cause of disability . . .

1.01 Category of Impairments, Musculoskeletal

1.03 Arthritis of a major weight-bearing joint (due to any cause):

With history of persistent joint pain and stiffness with signs of marked limitation of motion or abnormal motion of the affected joint on current physical examination. With a) Gross anatomic deformity of the hip or knee (e.g., subluxation, contracture, bony or fibrous ankylosis, instability) supported by X-ray evidence of either significant joint space narrowing or significant bony destruction and markedly limiting ability to walk and stand, or b) reconstructive surgery or surgical arthrodesis of a major weight bearing joint and return to full weight bearing status did not occur, or is not expected to occur within 12 months of onset.

1.04 Arthritis of one major joint in each of the upper extremities (due to any cause):

With history of persistent joint pain and stiffness, signs of marked limitation of motion of the affected joints on current physical examination, and X-ray evidence of either significant joint space narrowing or significant bony destruction. With a) abduction and forward flexion (elevation) of both arms at the shoulders, including scapular motion, restricted to less than 90 degrees, or b) gross anatomic deformity (e.g., subluxation, contracture, bony or fibrous ankylosis, instability, ulnar deviation) and enlargement or effusion of the affected joints.

CAN TOTAL DISABILITY BE PREVENTED?

Working improves our esteem and self-worth. An enjoyable job is fulfilling and emotionally satisfying. For those motivated to work and determined to overcome the impairments of handicap, there are many strategies to employ. Is there a workplace modification which minimizes stress to a joint and decreases repetitive use injury? This might include handicapped parking, a raised toilet seat with adjacent bars for those with hip disease, or ergonomically acceptable stools, chairs, worktables, or computer workstations. Allowing employees to use ramps rather than stairs is also very useful for osteoarthritis patients.

It is important to be up-front and positive with your employer. Emphasize what you can do rather than what cannot be done. Explain how your productivity can be greatly increased with minimal and noncostly modifications. Can you do some of your work out of the house to minimize travel and mobility problems? Could an occupational therapy workstation evaluation improve your comfort level? Is vocational rehabilitation or job retraining a realistic option?

SUMMARY

It has been said that arthritis patients are not disabled, but "differently abled," and this positive approach towards impairments and handicaps will allow more people to maintain self-esteem and to work longer in a satisfying environment.

26

Prognosis

Well, now, there's a remedy for everything except death.
—Miguel de Cervantes (1547–1616)

Now that we know what osteoarthritis is, who develops the condition, and how it is manifested and treated, what happens to people with the disease? The outcome is influenced by how society approaches the condition as well as how patients view it. This chapter approaches the issue from the patient's point of view.

WHAT HAPPENS TO OSTEOARTHRITIS OVER TIME?

The prognosis of osteoarthritis is as variable as those afflicted with the condition. The outcome of secondary forms of osteoarthritis such as ochronosis, Wilson's disease, acromegaly, and hyperparathyroidism (detailed in chapter 9) is entirely dependent upon how they are managed. Successful treatment of the causes of these conditions can sometimes even prevent osteoarthritis from occurring.

For all practical purposes, the outcome of generalized osteoarthritis depends on location. Which joints are affected, and to what degree? Osteoarthritis takes years to evolve, and joint pain does not closely correlate with radiographic signs of joint degeneration. In contrast, by the time a cardiac patient has chest pain or a heart attack, the coronary arteries have been diseased for years. Let's go on a quick tour of the body to look at how regional problems might affect prognosis.

Knee osteoarthritis

The prognosis of knee osteoarthritis runs the gamut. Some individuals go along for years with very little progression, while others progress very quickly and require a knee replacement within very few years. If the disease advances, the scenario below applies.

In general, the prognosis relates to how much articular cartilage is left in the joint. Loss of articular cartilage results in joint pain when walking on a flat surface, and leads to difficulties performing daily physical activities such as climbing up stairs, lowering into or rising from a chair, or getting in and out of the bathtub. If a X-ray demonstrates loss of the articular cartilage, then more loss is likely. We do not yet know all the things that contribute to the progression of articular cartilage loss and the need for joint replacement. We also do not yet know which treatments or exercises are effective in preventing the progression of knee osteoarthritis.

When knee osteoarthritis is initially diagnosed, the pain can usually be treated with exercises, analgesics, and anti-inflammatory medications. Within a few years, however, it often becomes more painful to walk for more than a block on a flat surface, the knee gets stiff when you sit for long periods, and it may swell after a lot of activity. As knee osteoarthritis gets worse, the joint may remain swollen all the time, and any walking will be painful. The quadriceps muscle above the knee can become smaller and weaker.

At some point, a physician may inject steroids into the knee to help reduce swelling and pain. This can be done about three times a year. You may need a cane when walking to provide assistance in balance, or to protect the painful knee. The physician may also prescribe a stronger pain medication such as a narcotic analgesic to help when knee pain becomes more severe. When an X-ray shows that there is very little cartilage left and your ability to do any physical activity is markedly reduced, it is time to consider a total joint replacement.

The rate at which a knee joint degenerates is highly variable. Studies suggest that advanced age, continued heavy weight-bearing activities such as running, other weight-bearing activities or physical labor that require bending and kneeling, abnormal angulations of the knee, increased weight, and low blood levels of vitamin D may also increase the rate of progression. Studies also show that low-impact exercises such as yoga, water aeorbics, and quadriceps strengthening may improve or reduce joint pain. However, we have no data demonstrating that these exercises reduce the rate of further cartilage degeneration.

Hip osteoarthritis

We know less about the prognosis of hip osteoarthritis than we do about the knee, even though it is one of the most common areas of involvement. Hip joint degeneration occurs at a rather early age (around 40) in individuals born with abnormal geometry of the hip such as dysplasias of either the acetabulum or the femur. These congenital abnormalities result in hip osteoarthritis from an abnormal hip joint at an early age (see chapter 24).

For individuals who develop hip disease later in life, the outcome can be favorable or progressive. As with knee osteoarthritis, the degree of joint degeneration depends on the rate of articular cartilage loss. Pain from hip osteoarthritis is highly individualized in that a person can experience pain with very little joint space loss or when the joint space is nearly gone. Generally, as hip disease worsens, walking becomes painful and the hip is painful at night. Use of pain medications and a cane can help for a while, but over time the pain becomes worse and the hip joint needs to be replaced.

The rate in which hip osteoarthritis progresses is not well-known. The few studies performed suggest that weight-bearing activities and physical labor increase the rate of joint degeneration in the hip. Low blood levels of vitamin D are also associated with hip joint degeneration. However, unlike knee osteoarthritis, patients with hip disease usually come to their doctor with a more advanced form of osteoarthritis and pain. Therefore, it is often just a matter of a year or two before they require a joint replacement. Studies performed in Europe found that nearly 60% of patients had a hip replacement within one or two years of first seeing their physician.

Hand osteoarthritis

Heriditary nodal osteoarthritis—the common form of hand osteoarthritis that develops in women around age 50—results in bony enlargement around the distal and proximal knuckles of the hands. While these women (or men), have knobby knuckles and may not like the way their hands appear, except for some stiffness and occassional pain, their prognosis is good. The joints develop bony enlargments and the fingers can feel stiff, but they usually do not become markedly deformed, remain functional, and do not progress to the point where a joint replacement is necessary.

Osteoarthritis can develop in the joint that connects the wrist to the base of the thumb. Seen mostly in women, this type of arthritis becomes painful and results in trouble writing or typing for any period of time. The pain can usually be controlled with analgesics, anti-inflammatories, splinting, and corticosteroid injections. Occasionally the pain becomes severe enough that surgery is required to try to realign or replace the joint.

Osteoarthritis of the feet and ankles

Although any part of the foot can be involved, most osteoarthritis problems are found at the great toe (MTP) joint. Usually the discomfort can initially be controlled with pain medications and by proper footwear or orthotics. A metatarsal bar can be put on the outside of the shoe to decrease stress on the arthritic joint. Over time, pain can become worse and an injection of corticosteroid may be helpful in reducing its intensity. In general, individuals with osteoarthritis of the first MTP joint adapt well and function fairly normally. If the pain is severe and is not controlled by pain medications, and toe deformities prevent you from wearing normal shoes, replacement surgery of the first MTP joint may be necessary. This procedure is usually performed by a podiatrist or an orthopedic surgeon.

Osteoarthritis of the ankle is uncommon. However, individuals who have sustained ankle trauma (such as a number of ankle sprains or broken bones) do have an increased risk of developing osteoarthritis in that joint. Individuals usually experience pain while walking and have some swelling, which is usually controlled with anti-inflammatory medications, pain medications, and sometimes an ankle support. If the pain is very severe, not controlled by medication, and limits activity, surgery may be advisable. Usually an ankle fusion is done to stabilize the joint. There are no satisfactory total ankle replacements at this time.

Osteoarthritis of the spine

Spinal disc degeneration usually starts when we are young adults. However, the chronic back pain associated with spinal disc degeneration does not normally bother us until our forties. As with any back pain, it usually comes and goes, and flares of pain are associated with increased activity or lifting heavy objects. Usually the pain can be controlled with pain medications, occasional bedrest, and epidural injections of corticosteroids, if necessary. If the osteoarthritic process becomes very severe and limits the ability to walk, the diagnosis of spinal canal stenosis (the narrowing of the spinal canal, causing nerve root symptoms and severe pain) or a herniated disc should be considered, and a surgical procedure may be required to clean out the extra bone. In general, individuals with spinal disc degeneration experience flare-ups of their disease a number of times during a year, but these episodes are usually somewhat self-limited and can be managed conservatively.

Osteoarthritis of the shoulder

Shoulder osteoarthritis is uncommon. Most cases result from sports-related or other traumatic injuries. In general, shoulder osteoarthritis can be managed conservatively with pain medications and occasional corticosteroid injections. Severe pain that cannot be controlled with medications may require a local procedure (such as arthroscopy) or a total joint replacement. Total shoulder replacement surgery is associated with a general reduction in pain, but also a limited range of motion.

SUMMARY

Osteoarthritis of the hip and knee have the worst prognosis, from the standpoint of the likelihood of needing aggressive therapy. Back, hand, and foot pain is usually self-limited and can be treated with medication, physical measures, and supports. Osteoarthritis of the shoulder and ankle are uncommon and usually occur after injuries to the area. And now for the good news: there are many promising new approaches to osteoarthritis on the horizon. Have a look at the next chapter.

27

New Directions

Is There Hope for a Cure?

*We're all of us guinea pigs in the laboratory of God. Humanity
is just a work in progress.*
—Tennessee Williams (1911–1983)

The standard treatments for osteoarthritis available today include non-pharmacologic and pharmacologic remedies. Nonpharmacologic therapies involve losing weight, exercising to improve muscle strength and endurance, and improving an overall sense of well-being. Drug treatments include pain and anti-inflammatory medications as well as corticosteroid injections. Surgical and complementary approaches have also been reviewed. Despite these often effective treatments, osteoarthritis is associated with an unacceptably high risk of causing loss of function and disability, and with poor self-esteem and societal dependency. Fortunately, researchers are looking into a variety of creative and innovative therapies. This chapter will review some of these promising avenues.

MAKING WHAT WE ALREADY HAVE, BETTER

The introduction of selective cox-2 blocking drugs in 1998 was a major step in making arthritis therapy effective and safer. Newer selective cox-2 blockers and related cox-3 and nitric oxide inhibitors will be on the market in the next few years. Tramadol (Ultram) blocks the excitatory amino acid pathway, which may be an important mediator of osteoarthritis as well as fibromyalgia pain. Newer-generation tramadols with improved analgesic properties should be available in the near future.

NEW FAMILIES OF MEDICINES

Metalloproteinase enzymes are released by chondrocytes and chew up articular cartilage. Blocking these enzymes with a metalloproteinase inhibitor represents a promising approach. Tetracycline antibiotics have metalloproteinase inhibiting properties as well as modest anti-arthritic effects.

Cytokines, small proteins released when the body is stressed or inflamed, act as hormones in that they signal cells to perform certain functions. Interleukin-1 (IL-1) is a cytokine that signals chondrocytes to increase the production of metalloproteinase enzymes. Several companies are testing IL-1 blockers for rheumatoid arthritis and their use in osteoarthritis represents an exciting potential approach.

Growth factors can stimulate chondrocyte cells to make more cartilage. Insulin growth factor-1 (IGF-1) stimluates cartilage growth in animals and is being looked at in humans. Other growth factors being looked at include insulin growth factor-2 and transforming growth factor-beta.

PROMISING SURGICAL OPTIONS

In early osteoarthritis, there are often small holes in the cartilage. These defects expand with time. Cartilage can be specially harvested from a non-weight-bearing area in the knee and placed into a small hole on the weight-bearing surface of the knee. This form of cartilage transplantation probably works best in young patients who have had a traumatic sports injury, but is of limited value in older individuals.

The outside of the bone (the periosteum) can also be moved to a small hole in the cartilage. Bone cells actually grow cartilage rather than bone. This type of bone transplantation has been performed for years with mixed success, but newer technologies are being explored to see if periosteum can be induced to make cartilage for a long period of time.

Cartilage-like material is a "biomaterial" that provides shock absorption and is being implanted into osteoarthritic joints. Some synthetic cartilage candidate biomaterials being studied include gel forms of type 1 collagens, gels of hyaluronan, and fibrin glues. Nonbiologic matrices consisting of felts of carbon fibers or polytetrafluoroethylene can have cartilage-like actions and are also being studied.

SUMMARY

In the next ten years, currently available families of medicines will be made safer and more effective, new families of medicines will be introduced, and our orthopedic colleagues will be able to create new, partially artificial musculoskeletal elements that will allow osteoarthritis patients more independence and the ability to function with less pain.

Glossary

acupuncture: traditional Chinese treatment for pain where very fine needles are inserted just under the skin at points along "life force" pathways called meridians

acute: of short duration and coming on suddenly

aerobic: an activity designed to increase oxygen consumption by the body

analgesic: a medication that decreases pain

arthritis: inflammation of a joint; generally perceived as any condition which involves the joints, cartilage, or bone

arthodesis: surgical fusion of a joint

arthroplasty: surgical reconstruction of a joint

arthroscopy: surgical evaluation and treatment of joint disease through an operating microscope

aspiration: the removal of fluid from a joint

biofeedback: control of unconscious biological functions such as pulse, respirations, blood pressure, and pain through a conscious thought process

Bouchard's nodes: nodal deformity of the second set of knuckles of the hands due to osteoarthritis

bunion: deformity of the great toe

bursa: a sac of synovial fluid between tendons, muscles, and bones that promotes easier movement; when inflamed, it causes a condition known as *bursitis*

capillaries: small blood vessels connecting the arteries to veins

capsaicin: a cayenne pepper derivative that decreases pain when applied topically

carpal tunnel syndrome: a condition where compression of the median nerve as it traverses the palmar side of the wrist produces shooting pains in the fingers

cartilage tissue: the material that covers bone

chiropractic: a therapy involving manipulation of the spine and joints to influence the body's nervous system and natural defense mechanisms

chondroitin sulfate: part of a protein found in cartilage, which may improve osteoarthritis when given as a pill

chronic: persisting over a long period of time

collagen: structural protein found in bone, cartilage, and skin

complete blood count (CBC): a blood test that measures the amount of red blood cells, white blood cells, and platelets in the body

computerized axial tomography (CAT): a form of imaging of a region of the body using a specialized type of X-ray

corticosteroid: any anti-inflammatory hormone made by the adrenal gland's cortex

cortisone: a synthetic corticosteroid

costochondritis: irritation of the tethering tissues connecting the sternum to the ribs, producing chest pain (also called *Tietze's syndrome*)

cox-2 antagonists: selective nonsteroidal anti-inflammatory arthritis drugs which are better tolerated than nonselective drugs; examples include rofecoxib (Vioxx) and celeboxib (Celebrex)

cytokines: messenger chemicals of the immune system

degenerative joint disease: another term for osteoarthritis

disability: a limitation of function that compromises the ability to perform an activity within a range considered normal

dysfunction: partial, inadequate, or abnormal function of an organ tissue or system

edema: swelling, usually due to inflammation or fluid retention

electromyogram (EMG): a mapping of electrical activity within muscles; usually combined with a nerve conduction velocity, which can assess nerve damage or injury

enzyme: a protein that accelerates chemical reactions

epidemiology: the study of relationships between various factors that determine who gets a disorder and how many people have it

ergonomics: a discipline that studies the relationship between human factors, the design and operation of machines, and the physical environment

erythrocyte sedimentation rate: see sedimentation rate

estrogen: female hormone produced by the ovaries

exacerbation: symptoms reappear; a flare-up

fascia: a layer of tissue between the skin and muscle

fatigue: feeling weary or sleepy, with reduced efficiency of work, accomplishment, or concentration

fibromyalgia: chronic neuromuscular pain characterized by fatigue, sleep disorder, soft tissue tender points, and systemic symptoms

fibrositis: an old name for fibromyalgia (see above); discarded since it implies inflammation, which is usually not present

fibrous capsule: an outer layer of wrapping that includes tendons and ligaments surrounding a joint

gene: consisting of DNA, it is the basic unit of inherited information in our cells

glucosamine: a sugar that plays a role in cartilage production and repair; when taken as a pill with or without chondroitin sulfate, it may improve osteoarthritis

handicap: a physical limitation; something that cannot be done

Hebreden's nodes: nodal swelling or growths of the outer knuckles of the hand

heel spur: calcification of the plantar fascia at the base of the heel

homeopathy: a discipline based on the idea that symptoms can be eliminated by taking infinitesimal amounts of an irritant or infectious agent that in large amounts would produce full-blown illness

hormones: chemical messengers (including thyroid, steroids, insulin, estrogen, progesterone, and testosterone) made by the body

hyperalgesia: exaggerated response to a truly painful stimulus

hypermobility: laxity of ligaments allowing one to assume positions or undertake movements difficult for a normal person to do

hyaluronan: a sticky material found in normal joint fluid; acts as a shock absorber

impairment: an anatomic, physiological, or psychological loss that leads to disability

immunity: a body's defense against foreign substances

incidence: the rate at which a population develops a disorder

inflammation: swelling, heat, and redness resulting from the infiltration of white blood cells into tissues

isometrics: exercises that strengthen muscle without moving the joints

isotonics: exercises that strengthen muscle by moving the joints

joint: the articulation between two bones

ligament: a tether attaching bone to bone, providing stability

lymphadenopathy: a condition producing swollen, palpable lymph nodes

lymphocyte: type of white blood cell that fights infection and mediates the immune response

magnetic resonance imaging (MRI): a picture of a body region derived from using magnets; involves no radiation

methylmethacrlate cement: used by orthopedists to anchor prostheses to bone

muscle: a primary tissue consisting of specialized contractile cells

myalgia: pain in the muscles

myofascial pain: discomfort in the muscles and fascia

myofascial pain syndrome: fibromyalgia-like pain limited to one region of the body, also known as regional *myofascial pain*

narcotics: an opiate-derived substance that suppresses pain

National Institutes of Health: a federal organization that funds medical research

neurotransmitters: chemical substances that transmit messages through nerves

nociceptor: a nerve that receives and transmits painful stimuli; *nociception* is the process that transmits this from the periphery (skin, muscles, tissues) to the central nervous system

nonsteroidal anti-inflammatory drugs (NSAIDS): an agent such as aspirin, ibuprofen, or naproxen that fights inflammation by blocking the actions of prostaglandin

occupational therapy: an approach using ergonomics in designing tasks to fit the capabilities of the human body

opiates: narcotics

orthopedist: a doctor who operates on musculoskeletal structures

orthotics: corrective devices used in footwear to correct deformities and alleviate foot pain

osteoarthritis: a degenerative disease of the joints

osteoblasts: cells that form bone

osteoclasts: cells that resorb bone

osteophytes: bony growth at the margin of an osteoarthritic joint

osteopath: a physician who is trained in performing specialized physical manipulative modalities

osteoporosis: loss of calcium in normal bone

osteotomy: orthopedic procedure which involves cutting of bone

overuse syndrome: pain in the muscles, ligaments, tendons or joints from excessive activity

pain: an unpleasant sensation or emotional experience

paresthesia: a sensation of numbness, tingling, burning, or prickling

pathogenic: causing disease, or abnormal reactions

peripheral nervous system: nerves to and from the spinal cord that transmit sensation and motor reflexes

physiatrist: a practitioner of physical medicine

physical medicine: a physician specializing in the principles of musculoskeletal, cardiovascular, and neurologic rehabilitation

physical therapy: conducted by allied health professionals who assist patients with physical conditioning

placebo: a pill or treatment that has no physiologic actions

plasma: the fluid portion of blood

polymyalgia rheumatica: an autoimmune disease of the joints and muscles seen in older patients with high sedimentation rates who have aching in their shoulders, upper arms, hips, and upper legs

polymyositis: an autoimmune, inflammatory disorder of muscles

prevalence: how many people have a condition per unit of population

primary fibromyalgia syndrome: fibromyalgia of unknown cause

prostaglandin: physiologically active substances present in many tissues

protein: a collection of amino acids; antibodies are proteins

psychogenic rheumatism: complaints of joint pain for purposes of secondary gain

range of motion: the amount of flexion, extension, abduction, adduction, internal and external rotation of movement of a joint

Raynaud's phenomenon: discoloration of the hands or feet (they turn blue, white, or red) especially with cold temperatures; a feature of autoimmune disease

referred pain: pain perceived as coming from an area different from its actual origin

reflexology: a form of alternative medicine based on the theory that specific areas of the body correspond to organs, glands, and nerves

regional myofascial syndrome: fibromyalgia pain limited to one region of the body, also known as *myofascial pain syndrome*

remission: a period free from symptoms, but not necessarily indicative of a cure

repetitive strain syndrome: caused when repetitive motions in a work environment produce strain or stress on an area of the body (as in carpal tunnel syndrome from excessive typing)

restless legs syndrome: legs that suddenly shoot out, lift, jerk, or go into spasm; if this occurs while asleep, it is called *sleep myoclonus*

rheumatic disease: any of 150 disorders affecting the immune or musculoskeletal systems

rheumatism: old term used to denote any musculoskeletal condition

rheumatoid arthritis: chronic disease of the joints, marked by inflammatory changes in the joint lining membranes

rheumatologist: an internal medicine specialist who has completed at least a two year fellowship studying rheumatic diseases

sedimentation rate: test that measures the rate of fall of red blood cells in a column of blood; high rates indicate inflammation or infection

selective serotonin reuptake inhibitors: a class of drugs (such as Prozac) that treat depression and pain by boosting serotonin levels

serotonin: a chemical that aids sleep, reduces pain and influences mood and appetite, derived from tryptophan and stored in blood platelets

serum: clear liquid portion of the blood after removal of clotting factors

sign: an abnormal finding on a physical examination

soft tissue rheumatism: musculoskeletal complaints related to tendons, muscles, bursa, ligaments, and fascial tissues; includes fibromyalgia

spinal stenosis: a form of osteoarthritis of the spine where bone spurs point inward and compress the spinal cord

steroids: shortened term for corticosteroids, which are anti-inflammatory hormones produced by the adrenal gland's cortex, or synthetically

strain: injury to a muscle, tendon, or ligament

substance P: a neurotransmitter chemical that increases pain perception

sympathetic nervous system: a branch of the autonomic nervous system that regulates the release of norepinephrine

symptoms: a subjective complaint relating to a bodily function or sensation

syndrome: a constellation of associated symptoms, signs, and laboratory findings

synovium tissue: material that lines the joint; its removal is called a *synovectomy*

synovitis: inflammation of the tissues lining a joint

systemic: pertaining to or affecting the body as a whole

temporomandibular joint (TMJ) dysfunction syndrome: pain in the jaw joint associated with localized myofascial discomfort

tender point: an area of tenderness in the muscles, tendons, bony prominences, or fat pads

tendon: structure that attach muscle to bone; inflammation of it is termed *tendinitis*

Tietze's syndrome: another term for costochondritis

titer: amount of a substance

transcutaneous electric nerve stimulation (TENS): a form of electrical acupuncture used to alleviate musculoskeletal pain

tricyclic: a family of antidepressant drugs (such as Elavil) that relieve depression, promote restful sleep, relax muscles, and raise pain thresholds

trigger point: an area of muscle which, when touched, triggers a reaction of discomfort

urinalysis: analysis of a urine sample under the microscope

ultrasound: high-frequency sound waves transmitted as heat to alleviate musculoskeletal pain and spasm

vasculitis: inflammation of the blood vessels

viscosupplementation: injection of hyaluronan into a joint for therapeutic purposes

vocational rehabilitation training: reconfiguring an occupation (or determining a new one), taking into account one's educational background, physical skills, and any handicaps or impairments

yoga: maneuvers and positions which relax the body, mind, and breath

Appendix 2

Resources

Hundreds of articles, books, and websites were consulted in preparing this book. We did not intend to write a textbook laden with references, but rather an overview and summary which could provide the reader basic information about osteoarthritis. A few websites are cited in the text, and table 13 cites the American College of Rheumatology criteria for osteoarthritis of the hand, hip, and knee. For more information about osteoarthritis, see the listings below. Just about everything covered in this book can be found in these listings.

WHAT ARE THE BEST TEXTBOOKS THAT DEAL SPECIFICALLY WITH OSTEOARTHRITIS?

Moskowitz, Howell, Altman, Buckwalter, and Goldberg (Eds.), *Osteoarthritis: Diagnosis and Medical/Surgical Management*, 3rd edition WB Saunders, 2001.

Brandt, Doherty, and Lohmander, (Eds.), *Osteoarthritis*, Oxford University Press, 1998. Dr. Brandt has also written a pocket compendium, *Diagnosis and Nonsurgical Management of Osteoarthritis*, Professional Communications, Inc. 2000.

HOW CAN I FIND OUT MORE ABOUT ALTERNATIVE THERAPIES?

Horstman, *The Arthritis Foundation Guide to Alternative Therapies*, Arthritis Foundation, 1999.

Helpful websites:

Ask Dr Weil: *http://www.Drweil.com*

National Center for Complementary and Alternative Medicine, *http:// ncaam.nih.gov*, run by the National Institutes of Health

The Rosenthal Center for Complementary and Alternative Medicine, *http://cpmcnet.Columbia.edu/dept/rosentha*, run by Columbia University College of Physicians and Surgeons

WHAT ARE THE BEST RHEUMATOLOGY TEXTBOOKS?

Kelly et al. *Textbook of Rheumatology*, 6th edition (WB Saunders, 2000).

Koopman et al. *Arthritis and Allied Conditions: A Textbook of Rheumatology*, 14th edition (Lippincott Williams & Wilkins, 2001).

Klippel and Dieppe, *Rheumatology*, 2nd edition (Mosby, 2000).

Maddison, et al. *The Oxford Textbook of Rheumatology* (Oxford University Press, 1998).

ARE THERE PARTICULARLY HELPFUL COMPENDIUMS ABOUT OSTEOARTHRITIS FOR PRIMARY CARE PHYSICIANS AND ALLIED HEALTH PROFESSIONALS?

Primer on the Rheumatic Diseases, 12th edition, Arthritis Foundation, 2000.

Clinical Care in the Rheumatic Diseases, Association of Rheumatology Health Professional, 1996. Available from the American College of Rheumatology.

IF I WANT TO RAISE MONEY FOR ARTHRITIS RESEARCH, NEED INFORMATION ABOUT RHEUMATOLOGISTS, OR AM AN ARTHRITIS PATIENT, WHAT RESOURCES SHOULD I USE?

The Arthritis Foundation is the best patient resource and provides $20 million a year for arthritis research. *Contact information:* 1300 W. Peachtree Street, Atlanta, GA 30309-2904; 800-283-7800; www.arthritis.org.

Nearly all rheumatologists belong to the American College of Rheumatology. Its Research and Education Foundation spends $6 million a year funding research and rheumatology training programs. Contact information: 800 Century Place, Suite 250. Atlanta, GA 30045-4300; 404-633-377; www.rheumatology.org.

The U.S. government allocates about $250 million a year to the National Institute of Arthritis Muscuoloskeletal and Skin Diseases (NIAMS), of which less than 5% is spent on osteoarthritis research. A branch of the National Institutes of Health, it supports a resource service for rheumatic disease information. Contact information: Building 31, Room 4C05, 9000 Rockville Pike, Bethesda, MD 20892; www.nih.gov/niams/healthinfo.

WHAT OTHER BOOKS DO YOU RECOMMEND FOR ARTHRITIS PATIENTS?

Grelsamer and Loebl, *The Columbia Presbyterian Osteoarthritis Handbook* (Macmillan, 1996) is a well-written, patient-oriented book about osteoarthritis from an orthopedic prospective.

Lorig and Fries, *The Arthritis Helpbook* (first published twenty years ago and revised every two to three years) and *The Arthritis Foundation's Guide to Good Living with Osteoarthritis* (2000) are available from the Arthritis Foundation for those who want books written at a high school level.

SOURCES RELATED TO PARTICULAR CHAPTERS

Introduction: Why Write a Book on Osteoarthritis?

"Impact of arthritis and other rheumatic conditions on the health care system in the United States," 1997, *MMWR*, 1999; 48: 349–353.

Rao, Mihaliak, and Kroenke, et al., "Use of complementary therapies for arthritis among patients of rheumatologists." *Annals Intern Med*, 1999; 131: 409–416.

Chapter 1: What Is Osteoarthritis?

Altman, Asch, Bloch, et al., Development of criteria for the classification and reporting of osteoarthritis: classification of osteoarth-ritis of the knee," *Arthritis Rheum*, 1986; 1039–1049.

Altman, Alarcon, Appelrough, et al., "The American College of Rheumatology criteria for the classification and reporting of osteoarthritis of
the hand," *Arthritis Rheum*, 1990; 33: 1601–1610.

Altman, Alarcon, Appelrough, et al., "The American College of
Rheumatology criteria for the classification and reporting of osteoarthritis of the hip," *Arthritis Rheum*, 1991; 34: 505–514.

Chapter 2: The History of Osteoarthritis

Benedek, "Historical vignette: When did osteoarthritis become osteoarthritis?," *J Rheumatology*, 1999; 26: 1374–1376.

McCarty, *Landmark Advances in Rheumatology*, American Rheumatism
Association, 1984.

Chapter 3: Who Gets Osteoarthritis?

Mc Alindon, Felwon, Zhang, et al., "Relationship of dietary intake and
serum levels of vitamin D to progression of osteoarthritis of the knee
among participants in the Framingham study," *Annals Intern Med*,
1996; 125: 353–359.

Spector, Cicuttini, Baker, Genetic influences on osteoarthritis in women:
a twin study, *Brit Med J*, 1996; 312: 940–945.

Sandmark, Higstedt, Lewold, et al., "Osteoarthritis of the knee in men
and women in association with overweight, smoking and hormone
therapy," *Annals Rheum Dis*, 1999; 58: 151–155.

Chapter 4: Bone

Meulenbelt, Bijkerk, Miedema, "A genetic association study of the IGF-1
gene and radiological osteoarthritis in a population-based cohort
study," *Annals Rheum Dis*, 1998; 57: 371–374.

Dewire, Einhorn, "The joint as an organ," in *Osteoarthritis: Diagnosis
and surgical management*, 3rd edition, Moskowitz, et al. (eds.), WB
Saunders, Philadelphia, PA, 2001, 49–68.

Chapter 5: Cartilage and Its Accomplices

Sah, Chen, Chen, et al., *Articular cartilage repair*, Koopman (ed.), *Arthritis and Allied Conditions*, 15th Edition, Lippincott Williams & Wilkins,
Philadelphia, PA, pp 2264–2278, 2000.

Buckwalter, Mankin, "Articular cartilage: degeneration and osteoarthritis: Repair, regeneration and transplantation," *Arthritis Rheum*, 1998;
41: 1331–1442.

Chapter 6: What Causes Osteoarthritis?

Felson, Anderson, Naimark, et al., "Obesity and knee arthritis: The Framingham Study," *Ann Int Med*, 1988; 109; 18–24.

Poole, Howell, "Etiopathogenesis of osteoarthritis, in Osteoarthritis: Diagnosis and Medical/Surgical Management," Moskowitz (ed.) et al., 3rd edition, WB Saunders, Philadelphia, PA, 2001, 29–48.

Chapter 7: What Happens at a Musculoskeletal Examination?

Polley and Hunder, "Rheumatologic Interviewing and Physical Examination of the Joints," WB Saunders, 1978.

Liang and Sturrock, "Evaluation of musculoskeletal symptoms," in *Rheumatology*, Klippel and Dieppe (eds.), Mosby, 1994.

Chapter 8: How is Osteoarthritis Diagnosed?

Sack, "Topics in primary care medicine: Osteoarthritis: A continuing challenge," *West J Med*, 1995; 163: 579–586.

O'Reilly and Doherty, "Signs, symptoms, and laboratory tests," in *Osteoarthritis*, Brandt, Doherty, and Lohmander (eds.), Oxford University Press, 1998.

Chapter 9: The Many Faces of Osteoarthritis

Schumacher, "Secondary osteoarthritis," in *Osteoarthritis: Diagnosis and Medical/Surgical Management*, Moskowitz (ed.), WB Saunders, 2000.

Schumacher, Gordon, and Paul, et al., "Osteoarthritis, crystal deposition, and inflammation," *Semin Arthritis Rheum* 1981; 11: 116–119.

Chapter 10: How Can I Be Sure It's Really Osteoarthritis?

Balint and Szebenyi, "Diagnosis of osteoarthritis. Guidelines and current pitfalls," *Drugs* 1996; 52 (supp 3): 1–13.

Ehrlich, "Osteoarthritis beginning with inflammation; definitions and correlations," *JAMA*, 1975; 232: 175–179.

Chapter 11: The Upper Body and Extremities

Brandt, "Clinical features of osteoarthritis," in *Diagnosis and Nonsurgical Management of Osteoarthritis*, Brandt (ed.), Professional Communications, 1996.

Cunningham and Diepp, "Study of 500 patients with limb joint osteoarthritis. L Analysis by age, sex, and distribution of symptomatic joint sites," *Annals Rheum Dis* 1991; 50: 8–13.

Chapter 12: The Spine

Yoo and, Krupkin, "Lumbar Spine," in *Osteoarthritis: Diagnosis and Medical/Surgical Management,* 3rd edition, Moskowitz (ed.), WB Saunders, Philadelphia PA, 3rd edition, 587–635, 2001.

Felson, Lawrence, and Dieppe, et al., "Osteoarthritis: New Insights, Part 1, The disease and its risk factors," *Annals Intern Med* 2000; 133: 635-646.

Chapter 13: The Lower Body

Klapper and Huey, *Heal Your Hips,* John Wiley & Sons, 1999.

Massardo, Watt, Cushnaghan, and Dieppe, "Osteoarthritis of the knee joint: an eight-year prospective study," *Annals Rheum Dis,* 1989; 48: 893–897.

Michelson, "Lower extremity considerations: Foot and ankle," in *Osteoarthritis: Diagnosis and Medical/Surgical Management,* 3rd edition, Moskowitz (ed.), WB Saunders, 2001.

Chapter 14: You Can Conquer Osteoarthritis

McIlwain and Bruce, *Stop Osteoarthritis Now!,* Simon and Shuster, 1996.

Lorig, Lubeck, and Kraines, et al., "Outcomes of self-help education for patients with arthritis," *Arthritis Rheum,* 1985; 28: 680–685.

Lorig, Fries, and Gecht, *The Arthritis Helpbook. A tested self-management program for coping with your arthritis,* Perseus Press, 2000.

Chapter 15: Living Well with Osteoarthritis

The Arthritis Foundation's Guide to Good Living with Osteoarthritis, Arthritis Foundation, 2000.

Chapter 16: Exercises to Improve Osteoarthritis

The Arthritis Foundation's Guide to Good Living with Osteoarthritis, Arthritis Foundation, Atlanta, GA, 2000.

Lane, *Exercise: A cause of osteoarthritis?,* Rheum Dis Clin NA, 1993; 19: 617–633.

Ettinger Jr, Burns, Messier, "A randmonized trial comparing aerobic exercise and resistance exercise with a health education program," *JAMA,* 1997; 277: 25–31.

Chapter 17: How Osteoarthritis Medicines Are Tested

Altman, Brandt, Hochberg, et al., "Design and conduct of clinical trials in patients with osteoarthritis: recommendation from a task force of the Osteoarthritis Research Society," Osteoarthritis Cartilage 1996; 4: 217–243.

Chapter 18: Medicines that Work for Osteoarthritis

Griffin, Brandt, Liang, et al., "Practical management of osteoarthritis: integration of pharmacologic and nonpharmacologic measures," *Arch Fam Med*, 1995; 4: 1049–1055.

Bradley, Brandt, Katz, et al., "Comparison of an inflammatory dose of ibuprofen, an analgesic dose of ibuprofen and acetaminophen in the treatment of patients with osteoarthritis of the knee," *N Engl J Med*, 1991; 325: 87–91.

Hochberg, "Clinical features and treatment of osteoarthritis," *Primer on Rheumatic Diseases*, Arthritis Foundation, Atlanta, GA, 11th edition, pp 218–221.

Chapter 19: Local Medical Therapies

Felson, Lawrence, and Hochberg, et al., "Osteoarthritis: New Insights, Part 2, Treatment approaches," *Ann Intern Med*, 2000; 133: 726–737.

Brandt, Smith, and Simon, "Intraarticular injection of hyaluronan as treatment for knee osteoarthritis: What is the evidence?" *Arthritis Rheum*, 2000; 43: 1192–1203.

Chapter 20: But Doctor, I'm in Pain!

Bollet, "Edema of the bone marrow can cause pain in osteoarthritis and other diseases of bone and joints," *Annals Intern Med*, 2001; 134: 591–593.

Symmons, "Knee pain in older adults: the latest musculoskeletal epidemic," *Ann Rheum Dis*, 2001; 60: 89–90.

"The management of chronic pain in older persons: AGS Panel on Chronic Pain in Older Persons," American Geriatrics Society, *J Am Geriatric Soc*, 1998; 46: 635–651.

Chapter 21: When Do We Operate?

"Total hip replacement: NIH Concensus Development Panel on Total Hip Replacement," *JAMA*, 1995; 273: 1950–1956.

Lavernia, Guzman, and Gachupin-Garcia, "Cost effectiveness and quality of life for knee arthroplasty," *Clin Orthop*, 1997; 345: 134–139.

"Surgical Management of Osteoarthritis," in *The Columbia Presbyterian Osteoarthritis Handbook*, Grelsamer and Loebl (eds.), Macmillan, 1996.

Chapter 22: Alternative Therapies

Horstman, "Alternative Therapies," Arthritis Foundation, Atlanta, GA, 1999

Collinge, "American Holistic Health Association Complete Guide to Alternative Medicine," Warner Books, 1996.

Lorig, Holman, Lauren, et al., "Living a healthy life with chronic illness," California Bull Publications, Palo Alto, CA, 1994.

Chapter 23: I Have Osteoarthritis

Elders, "The increasing impact of arthritis on public health," *J Rheumatol* 2000; 27 (supp 60): 6–8.

What is a rheumatologist? Brochure, American College of Rheumatology, 1995.

Chapter 24: Special Cases

Schumacher, "Secondary osteoarthritis," in *Osteoarthritis: Diagnosis and Medical/Surgical Management*, 3rd edition, Moskowitz (ed.), WB Saunders, Philadelphia, PA, 3rd edition, 327–358, 2001.

Croft, Cooper, and Wickham, et al., "Osteoarthritis of the hip and acetabular dysplasia," *Annals Rheum Dis*, 1991; 50: 308–310.

Chapter 25: Can Or Should I Work?

Hadler, *Occupational Musculoskeletal Disorders*, 2nd edition, Lippincott Williams & Wilkins, 1999.

Social Security Guidelines for Disability, U.S. Government, Revised 1994, Disability Evaluation under Social Security.

Index

acetaminophen
  and causes of osteoarthritis, 19
  and history of osteoarthritis, 10
  as medication that works on
    osteoarthritis, 73, 78, 91, 102, 108,
    163–64, 165, 166, 168
  and pain, 178, 179, 180, 182
  and pregnancy, 206–8
  side effects of, 164
  and who gets osteoarthritis, 19
  and who treats osteoarthritis, 198
Achilles tendon, 114, 207
acromegaly, 57–58, 60, 217
acromioclavicular osteoarthritis, 73
activities of daily living (ADL), 43, 120–21,
    129, 135, 178, 201, 212, 218
acupressure/acupuncturists, 134, 202
African Americans, 13, 21
age
  and cartilage and associated tissues, 34
  and diagnosis of osteoarthritis, 62, 64
  and disability, 213
  and DISH, 95
  and history of joint injuries, 16–17
  and new directions for osteoarthritis,
    223
  and osteoarthritis of specific body part,
    78, 86, 87, 108
  and prognosis of osteoarthritis, 219
  and specialized forms of osteoarthritis,
    56
  and statistics about osteoarthritis, 4
  and surgery, 187

  and testing of medications, 161, 162
  and who gets osteoarthritis, 11, 13, 14,
    16–17, 18, 21
allied health professionals, 189, 201, 202
alternative therapies/practitioners, 191–96,
    208
American Academy of Orthopedic Sur-
    geons, 10
American College of Rheumatology, 6, 10,
    158, 161–62, 163–64, 165, 166
American Medical Association, 3
Americans with Disabilities Act, 214
"analgesic hip" syndrome, 19
analgesics, 19, 44, 156–57, 179, 180, 218, 220,
    223
anatomy, lesson about, 80–85
anemia, 43, 47, 48
anesthesia/anesthesiologists, 10, 178, 187,
    200
ankles, 45, 59, 112–15, 128, 130, 185, 187, 200,
    206, 220, 221. *See also* feet
ankylosing hyperostosis, 95
ankylosing spondylitis, 9, 42, 44, 48, 65, 85,
    86, 96, 121, 215
anti-inflammatory drugs
  and alternative therapies, 194, 195
  and causes of osteoarthritis, 19
  and diagnosis of osteoarthritis, 44
  and local medical therapies, 171, 173
  as medication that works on
    osteoarthritis, 74, 78, 92, 106, 115, 165
  and new directions for osteoarthritis,
    223

Social Security, 214, 215
social workers, 201
soft tissue, 6, 42–43, 49, 51, 57–58, 63, 65.
    See also fibromyalgia
South Africa, 54
soybean oils, 193–94
SPECT (single photon emission computed tomography), 51
speech pathologists, 199
Spender, John Kent, 3, 9
spinal cord, 59, 81, 84, 197
spinal stenosis, 51, 53, 88, 92, 94–95, 96, 97, 185, 200, 221
spine
    and anatomy lesson, 80–85
    construction and functions of, 30, 80–85, 95–96
    crooked, 91
    curvature of, 88, 205
    and diagnosis of osteoarthritis, 50
    and disability, 214–15
    and effects of osteoarthritis, 72
    and exercise, 149–50
    manipulation of, 200–1
    and menopause and hormones, 28
    and premature osteoarthritis, 205
    and prognosis of osteoarthritis, 221
    radicular symptoms of osteoarthritis of, 97
    and shoulders, 72
    and specialized forms of osteoarthritis, 57
    and who gets osteoarthritis, 20
    and who treats osteoarthritis, 199, 200–1
    See also back; neck
spinous processes, 84, 87
splints, 129, 130, 131, 136, 179, 201, 206, 220
spondylitis, 203
spondylolisthesis, 89, 91, 96
spondylosis, 89, 91, 96
sports. *See* athletes/sports
spurs. *See* bone spurs
Stanford University, 4, 17
sternal (breast bone) joints, 70–71
steroids, 58, 171–72, 173, 174, 180, 182, 208, 218
stiffness
    and alternative therapies, 195

in back and neck, 87, 95–96
and diagnosis of osteoarthritis, 42–43, 46, 62, 63, 64
and disability, 215
and DISH, 95
and exercise, 146
in hands, 161
in hips, 102
in knees, 108
and living with osteoarthritis, 129, 132
and prognosis of osteoarthritis, 218, 220
and testing of medications, 161, 162
stinging nettle, 195
Stone, Edmund, 10
strain, back and neck, 92, 97
strengthening, muscle, 20, 102, 108, 138, 139, 142–45, 146, 149–50, 206, 219, 222
Stuck, Walter, 10
subchondral bone, 27, 28
subchondral sclerosis, 27, 49, 58
substance P, 177, 194
support systems, 124–25, 183, 201, 213
supports. *See* assistive devices; *type of support*
surgery
    and assistive devices, 130
    and diagnosis of osteoarthritis, 44
    and disability, 215
    goals of, 185–86
    and history of osteoarthritis, 10
    and local medical therapies, 172
    and new directions for osteoarthritis, 223–24
    and outpatient procedures, 184–85
    and pain, 179, 180, 181, 182, 187–88
    and premature osteoarthritis, 205, 206
    and primer of orthopedic procedures, 185–86
    and prognosis of osteoarthritis, 220, 221
    side effects of, 188
    what can go wrong in, 188
    when to do, 183–88
    who should consider, 183–84
    and who treats osteoarthritis, 199, 200
    See also specific part of body
swelling
    and alternative therapies, 194
    in ankles, 220
    and causes of osteoarthritis, 38